The
LEAN
BODY
Promise

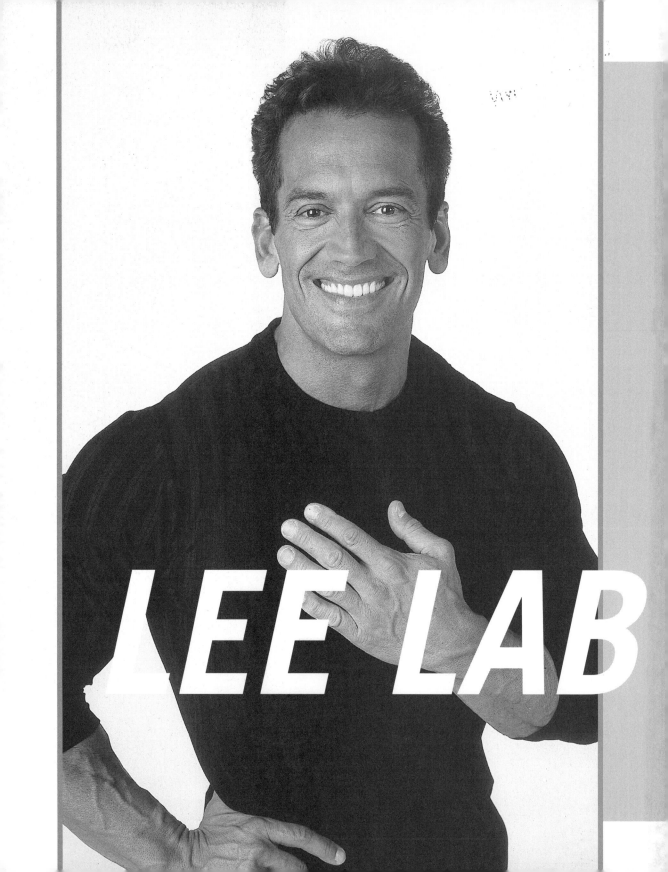

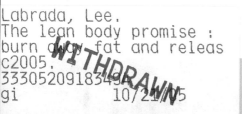

THE LEAN BODY Promise

RADA

BURN AWAY FAT

AND RELEASE THE

LEANER, STRONGER

BODY INSIDE YOU

Collins
An Imprint of HarperCollins Publishers
www.harpercollins.com

This book is written as a source of information only. The information contained in this book should by no means be considered a substitute for the advice of a qualified medical professional, who should always be consulted before beginning any new diet, exercise, or other health program.

This book has been carefully researched, and all efforts have been made to ensure the accuracy of its information as of the date published. All of the procedures, poses, and postures should be carefully studied and clearly understood before attempting them at home. The author and the publisher expressly disclaim responsibility for any adverse effects, damages, or losses arising from the use or application of the information contained herein.

HarperCollins books may be purchased for educational, business, or sales promotional use. For information please write: Special Markets Department, HarperCollins Publishers, 10 East 53rd Street, New York, New York 10022.

FIRST EDITION

Designed by William Ruoto

Library of Congress Cataloging-in-Publication Data has been applied for.

ISBN 0-06-059371-7

05 06 07 08 09   WBC/RRD   10 9 8 7 6 5 4 3 2 1

To my three sons, Hunter, Blade, and Pierce, with love

Contents

PART SIX: **Putting It All Together** **180**

Step #1: Make the Decision ❱ Step #2: Sign Your Name ❱ Step #3: Clean Out Your Fridge ❱ Step #4: Prepare Your Home Gym, or Join One ❱ Step #5: Schedule It ❱ Step #6: Do It ❱ Step #7: Savor the Results ❱ Step #8: Care and Maintenance of Your Lean Body ❱ Step #9: Stay in Touch with Your Lean Body Coach ❱ Step #10: Become a Fitness Evangelist ❱ My Lean Body Promise Letter

PART SEVEN: **Lean Body FAQs** **188**

Acknowledgments

This is an "action book" in which you are the "action hero." That's because once you read this book, you will be compelled to take certain actions that will change your life forever. That also makes this book about change—positive physical and mental change. This book is dedicated to all of you action heroes—those of you who will heed the call and embrace your potential for change. You will inspire others to do the same and will have a profound impact on many lives.

There's no such thing as a "self-made" man. Behind every successful human being is an entire supporting cast of individuals who have contributed their efforts along the way. I have been blessed richly with family, friends, and professional associates without whom this book would have merely been a passing idea. I want to thank you all.

To my mother, Maria, and father, Ele, who have selflessly dedicated their entire lives to the unconditional love and support of the Labrada family—I have no words that would adequately express my gratitude. Your courage, hard work, and discipline have left their indelible mark, inspiring me to fulfill my God-given potential. To my sisters, Conchita and Lourdes, my brother, Gene, and everyone in the Labrada and Valladares families—your unflagging love and support over the years have positively buoyed my spirits.

To my wife, Robin—I love you, beautiful woman. You are the wind beneath my wings and I wouldn't be where I am today without you. Thank you for your patience in reading through the numerous revisions of this book, and thank you for contributing the recipes—now others will be able to enjoy your home cooking also! To my sons, Hunter, Blade, and Pierce—thank you for being the finest bunch of boys a man could ever be blessed with. You guys always put a smile on my face, even on the tough days!

I wish to thank Joe Weider for building the sport of bodybuilding passionately and for providing a springboard for me and countless others; Arnold Schwarzenegger for the inspiration that he has provided me, as a fellow immigrant, bodybuilder, and businessperson; nutritionist Keith Klein for his mentoring and profound influence on my nutrition philosophies; Bill Phillips for giving me my start in the sports nutrition business and inspiring me to become a fitness evangelist; Dr. Tom Deters for coaching me during my early years as a competitive bodybuilder; and Craig DeSerf for being my loyal training partner and motivator over the years. There are many others, too many to name here, who have helped me; please know that in my heart I am grateful to you all.

I wish to extend special thanks to my writer, Duane Swierczynski, who did a fabulous job of capturing my "voice," assembling long hours of interviews, telephone conversations, and notes into a cohesive work of art—and kept his sense of humor through it all; my agent, David Hale Smith, for his wise guidance and for believing in me and the viability of *The Lean Body Promise* even when others didn't; Larry North for introducing us; Megan Newman for her faith in this project; and my reliable team at Labrada Nutrition (my "second family")—especially Christina Moreland and Gabe Canales—for their outstanding PR and marketing efforts, first on our Get Lean Houston! campaign and later on this book. I also want to thank Dr. Kyle Workman, Dr. Alan Zimmerman, Phil Kaplan, and Doug Kalman for reviewing my book and offering their helpful insights.

And what is an author without a first-class publishing team? I want to thank the entire crew at HarperCollins Publishers for their enthusiasm for and commitment to *The Lean Body Promise*. Special thanks to Stephen Hanselman, senior vice president and publisher, for his leadership; Greg Chaput, my editor, for embracing this book as if it were his and guiding me through its publication; Mary Ellen Curley, associate publisher; Shelby Meizlik, assistant director of publicity; and Josh Marwell, Nina Olmsted, and the rest of the sales team at Harper.

A great creative team is essential to the persona of a book. I want to thank Jay Rusovich for his outstanding photography, passion, and unyielding pursuit of the perfect picture; to Martin Shepeard for his direction and excellence in graphics; to Heather Robinson for gracing our pages with her fit, feminine form; and to Fit Gym in Houston, Texas, for the use of their first-rate facilities.

The
LEAN
BODY
Promise

The Promise

What if I told you that no matter what condition you are in now, I could show you how to make lifelong improvements in appearance, strength, self-image, and confidence in just 30 minutes each day?

It doesn't matter whether you are old or young, male or female, totally deconditioned or active; *you have the power to improve yourself*. And I can teach you how to do it.

Here's the promise that I want to make to you, and one that you must believe:

> **There is a strong, lean body inside you, and you have the power to release it.**

The Lean Body Promise is a 30-minute exercise, five-meal-a-day program that will dramatically transform your body in as few as 12 weeks. It's the ultimate fat solution, and the last get-in-shape program you'll ever need.

My program is based on the principle I call *Banex*, which stands for "balanced nutrition and exercise." Now, you've always heard that eating right and exercise are the way to get in shape and control your weight. But Banex takes this simple idea to the next level. With this revolutionary program, you'll eat more than ever before, in a way that boosts your metabolism and melts fats. With the power and cardio workouts, you'll receive the maximum results from a very short workout.

After reading this book, you'll be able to . . .

- Strengthen your heart and lungs, burn body fat, and build muscle
- Switch your body from "fat-storing" to "fat-burning" mode
- Eat the same delicious food you're accustomed to and crave
- Enjoy more food while burning more fat
- Build a stronger, leaner you in just 30 minutes a day
- Track your progress easily and accurately without a mirror or scale
- Achieve and enjoy the leaner, stronger, healthier body you desire and deserve

And it doesn't matter if you've failed to get into shape before. You can handle this program, no matter what shape you're in, no matter how many diets you've started and failed. I can show you how to get motivated—and stay motivated—so that you will succeed this time. You can forget about past failures. Just as you can build your body, you can build your willpower and leave your old self-destructive habits behind.

With the Lean Body Promise, it's not unusual to see dramatic changes within a few short weeks. Not only will your appearance improve, but you will also experience greater energy levels, and with that your spirits and motivation to make greater improvements will soar. The quality of your life will improve, and your success will have a profound, positive impact first on you, and then on everything else—your relationships with your family and friends, your workplace, and even society as a whole. It's what I call the "ripple effect."

I'll also show you how to measure your body fat so you'll be able to monitor your Lean Body as it emerges. In Appendix D (page 208) you'll find detailed instructions on how to track how much lean muscle you're building, and how much fat you're melting away.

Anyone can benefit from using the Banex principle. In the next part, you will find real-world examples of ordinary people who experienced extraordinary, life-transforming changes in their bodies by applying the principles in this book. You don't have to be an exercise physiologist or nutritional scientist to make sense of it. The Lean Body program is simple and effective, and fits into busy lifestyles.

I should know: I'm a full-time dad, husband, and president of a growing company. Yet it's easy to fit the simple guidelines of the Lean Body Promise into my life every day, even when it seems that the phone never stops ringing, the meetings never end, and I'm busy guiding my boys through the trials of long division.

The fact is, everything in this program is based on tried-and-tested principles that I have learned over the last 25 years in training myself and thousands of students, and from my work with professionals in the fields of nutrition and exercise. The Lean Body Promise has also been reviewed by experts in medicine, nutrition, exercise physiology, and chiropractic.

The Lean Body Promise is not a quick fix; it's even better. The Lean Body Promise is a practical system that you can easily make a part of your daily routine. It all starts with a 12-week personal improvement challenge. Then, it will become your own personal journey of physical self-improvement, keep you on track, and give you positive, lifelong habits and empowerment.

If you put your trust in me, I will help you to help yourself and you will succeed in transforming yourself. I will show you everything you need to know, and I will teach you how to keep yourself motivated.

So why trust *me*?

Helping Houston Get Lean

"That is *not* true!" I said, looking into the camera.

I was sitting alone in a television studio in Houston, Texas. Although I could not see my CNN *Crossfire* hosts and the other guest on the show, author Marilyn Wann, I knew that millions of people were watching me. *Crossfire* is known for its lively debate, and this evening's show had already become particularly animated.

Wann, the author of *Fat! So?* was joined by *Crossfire* host Tucker Carlson on one side of the discussion. I was on the other side with former Clinton campaign strategist Paul Begala. The debate topic: Should the government sponsor programs to educate people about obesity?

Ms. Wann had just made the assertion that "weight is highly genetic."

As Houston's recently appointed fitness czar, I knew that this was a comment I couldn't leave unaddressed. The future of overweight people watching the show that evening could very well hang in the balance. What if people left the show thinking that they were just naturally fat and there wasn't anything they could do to change their condition? There would be many who would use this as justification to give up on themselves.

As soon as the words shot out of my mouth—*"That is not true!"*—I launched into an explanation. "If weight was a genetic factor," I said, "then how could obesity amongst our young be up threefold in the last 20 years?"

I'm no geneticist, but common sense tells me that 20 years is not long enough for the American people to evolve—or mutate, if you prefer—into a race of fatsos. It's true that obesity is on the rise in the United States. But for the most part, this phenomenon can be attributed to lifestyle factors. People are becoming more overweight because they are eating more and exercising less.

This is deadly serious business. According to figures released by the Centers for Disease Control and Prevention (CDC), more than 300,000 deaths per year can be attributed to obesity-related causes. Obesity leads to an increased risk for life-threatening diseases including diabetes, cancer, and heart disease.

"Look, I'm only here to help," I explained.

The 5-foot, 4-inch, 270-pound Ms. Wann shot back: "I don't need your *help*."

Fair enough. Maybe she was irritated that I would offer to help her—or anyone else who is overweight—on national TV. But driving home, I couldn't help but wonder about the multitude of people who are needlessly battling a weight problem every day. And those who have thrown in the towel and given up hope of ever getting in shape.

It bugged me. Because I knew the answer to America's weight problem was as simple as making a promise to yourself.

You might be asking yourself: Okay, who went and appointed me "fitness czar," anyway? My appointment was brought on (in part) by *Men's Fitness* magazine, which named Houston "America's Fattest City" two years in a row. Now, that *really* bugged me.

Being the CEO and founder of Labrada Nutrition, a Houston-based Inc. 500 company in 2002, I caught a lot of ribbing from friends, both inside and outside of the sports nutrition industry. After all, I am in the business of getting people into shape. They knew Houston's unflattering title would get under my skin, and they rubbed it in. So I decided to do something about it.

America's Fattest Cities, 2002
(AS PER *MEN'S FITNESS* MAGAZINE)

1. **HOUSTON, TX**
2. Chicago, IL
3. Detroit, MI
4. Philadelphia, PA
5. Dallas, TX

With the help of my team at Labrada Nutrition, I formulated a citywide initiative that would raise awareness among Houstonians about the need to exercise and eat healthy in order to lose weight and get fit. The plan called for me to lead the charge. Given the opportunity, I knew that we could get the word out and educate people.

Happily, Houston's mayor, Lee Brown, agreed with me. A few months later, I arrived early at city hall and greeted my family, friends, and staff. I looked around the room and saw the media scurrying about, setting up cameras. Mayor Lee Brown took the microphone, announced the launch of the Get Lean Houston! campaign, and named me as the city's first fitness czar.

And that's when it happened. The magnitude of my mission took on a whole new meaning. I had a huge responsibility on my hands.

How can I get through to people so they can make lasting changes in their bodies? I asked myself.

Which made me think: *Well, how did* I *do it?*

25 Years in the Making

I've been an avid bodybuilder and fitness coach for over two decades, and during 10 of those years, I was ranked as one of the top four bodybuilders in the world. Some people have a preconception of bodybuilders as "gym rats," but my bodybuilding experience has actually helped me to develop simple exercise and nutrition techniques that anybody can use to make changes in their bodies they would have never thought possible.

These techniques are at least 25 years in the making. Let me show you where it all began.

I emigrated from Cuba to the United States with my grandmother when I was two years old, around the time of the Cuban missile crisis. My dad was trained as a civil engineer—he knew some English, not a lot. But within a month, he had landed a job as a civil engineer and proceeded to carve out a middle-class living for us. We settled in Chicago.

One of my earliest memories as a kid is walking down the beach on Lake Michigan. I would suck up my chest, stick out my ribs, and walk around like Steve Reeves from the *Hercules* movies. People would stare at me, and I loved the attention. Looking back, I think they were feeling sorry for me. *Look at this kid—he must be malnourished! You can see his ribs poking through!*

Not long after, I began sneaking into my dad's bedroom to mess around with his weightlifting set, and soon I was seeing changes in my arms. We had moved to Jacksonville, Florida, by that time, and I remember that I could always do more push-ups and sit-ups than any other kid in the entire apartment complex. People probably still thought I was malnourished.

By the time I was 16, I was working out every afternoon with a high school classmate. I kept working out every day after school, trying to get big. But my diet didn't support all of the crazy exercise I was doing. I had a fast metabolism, and while I was getting more muscular, more defined, I wasn't getting any bigger. I couldn't figure out why I wasn't turning into Steve Reeves—but there I was, eating bologna sandwiches.

I didn't know it then, but I was overtraining and not eating right.

There was a kid at my high school who was considered sort of an oddball at the time because he was a competitive bodybuilder. He was a lot bigger than I was, and I was curious as to how he got that way. I remember going up to him and asking him, "What's that weird stuff you drink out of your thermos every day?"

The young man turned to look at me, and for a second there, I thought he was going to knock my block off. Instead, he gave me an answer: milk mixed with protein and brewer's yeast. I started asking more questions, and as he patiently gave me answers, I was enthralled.

He also told me something else: There was another Mr. Jacksonville contest coming up in just four weeks. Now at this point, I was still a buck thirty, dripping wet. But I was also curious. I learned that the promoter of the contest was Jim Nelson, owner of a bodybuilding gym in Jacksonville and one of the top bodybuilders in Florida. The next day, I drove down to meet him at his gym, and at first I was stunned. I'd never seen a guy with that much muscle up close.

I signed the paperwork, then went back and trained like mad for a month at a place we fondly called "Griner's Gym." It was nothing more than a 15 by 15 wooden shack behind the house of a tough Jacksonville cop, Sergeant Jim Griner. Even though Sgt. Griner's gear was archaic by today's standards, it had everything I needed. In four weeks, I whipped myself into shape.

The morning of the competition I went in for prejudging and saw my competition backstage, warming up. I almost turned around and went home. These guys were at least 30 to 40 pounds bigger than I was—and those were the teenagers. I thought I didn't have a prayer. But somehow, I convinced myself to stay.

When the results came back that evening, not only had I won first place, but I had also won the "most muscular" trophy.

I was graduated from high school in 1978 and decided to attend Northwestern University. I remember going to orientation with my dad late that summer. We went to check out the school gym. Back then, it was nothing more than a Universal machine, an old, rickety wooden leg press, a bunch of weight plates strewn everywhere, and some benches. That was it. At first, I didn't think I'd be able to train there.

But I soon found that I could work out just as well at the Northwestern gym. This taught me an important lesson: you don't need a lot of fancy equipment to achieve good results. Anybody can take the basics—a set of good free weights and a solid bench—and shape his or her body as well as anyone with a million-dollar setup.

In 1979, my family moved to Houston, Texas, and I transferred to the University of Houston to be closer to them and finish my degree in civil engineering. Three years later, I began entering bodybuilding competitions once again, resulting in wins at the NPC (National Physique Committee) Collegiate Texas Championship, NPC Gulf Coast Classic, and NPC Texas State Championships. I went on to win my class at the 1985 NPC National Championships, and two weeks later I was crowned IFBB (International Federation of Bodybuilding) Mr. Universe at the ripe old age of 25.

That was the beginning of a string of professional bodybuilding wins, during which I was ranked as one of the top four bodybuilders in the world for seven consecutive years. In 2004, I was inducted into the IFBB Pro Bodybuilding Hall of Fame.

What was the key to my success? Knowing my body. I can eat something and know exactly how it'll affect me. As a pro bodybuilder, I had to know exactly how food, drink, stress, time changes—even the cabin pressure in an airplane—would affect the way I looked. Being smaller than most of my competitors, I couldn't afford to screw up. If I came in just 2 or 3 percent off, they'd trounce me. This is how I became so attuned to how foods affect the body, and how certain types of power and cardio workouts can quickly burn fat and build lean muscle.

In other words, I've been experimenting in my own personal lab—my body—for 25 years. Now I'm proud to share the results with you.

The Birth of the Lean Body Promise

Eventually, as my bodybuilding career drew to a close, my sister Conchita and I opened a personal training studio called Star Bodies in Houston. At its peak, we had 40 personal trainers working for us, who performed hundreds of personal training sessions per week for our clients. Then I went on to launch the company that I own and run today, Labrada Nutrition (www.labrada.com), which markets nutritional supplements and functional foods that help people stay in their best physical shape. I've used nutritional supplements all my life—hey, they work—and I felt that I could do a better job serving my customers than existing sports nutrition companies.

More importantly, Labrada Nutrition became the forum from which I would spread my message of Banex—balanced nutrition and exercise. I wanted to share my knowledge and educate others. I wanted them to enjoy the strong, lean body they never thought was possible.

My ability to spread this message made a quantum leap with the creation of the *Lean Body Coaching Club*, a free weekly e-newsletter. Suddenly, I was able to reach hundreds of people every week, instantly. I shared my ideas about exercise, nutrition, supplementation, fat burning—everything that I thought would help people get into better shape. And at the end of each e-mail, I'd include an encouraging word or two.

I started receiving e-mails from people thanking me. Some would tell me that they were about to skip their workout when they got my message, and that it had turned their day around.

The more words of encouragement, the more the e-mails would pour in. The *Lean Body Coaching Club* membership grew into hundreds of subscribers, went into thousands, and then into tens of thousands, purely by word of mouth.

The Revelation

One early winter morning, I was writing my weekly LBC e-newsletter when a news-flash came through my e-mail that would alter the course of my mission. It was the announcement that Houston had been named America's Fattest City by *Men's Fitness* magazine.

But what if this setback to the city's image could be turned into a positive opportunity to help people get lean and healthy?

Several months later, Get Lean Houston! was born, my appointment as fitness czar was official, and my mission was about to rocket to a new level. I decided to make a Get Lean Houston! program available free to anyone who wanted to download it from the Internet. I wrote a program that anyone could use to lose fat, tone muscle, and get in shape.

I witnessed large numbers of well-intentioned people come in with their New Year's resolutions each January. By March, most of the New Year's crowd had dropped out, and the gym population would be back to normal. Again I began to wonder why it was that some succeeded, but most failed.

After all, everyone had signed up for a gym membership and had begun a bona fide workout program written out by one of the club's instructors. They had actually taken their first steps. But somewhere along the way, most had lost their mojo.

The Two Reasons That People Fail

People embark on a get-in-shape program with the intention of changing for the better, but fail for two reasons: they lack the correct information, and they are unable to get motivated and stay motivated. These are the two biggest obstacles to lasting success in achieving and enjoying the leaner, stronger, healthier body you desire and deserve.

Let's take a look at each of these two reasons, and then let's see what we're going to do to address them. After all, you're reading this book because you think you want to change, right?

Reason #1: You've Got the Wrong Map

Let's say that I called you up one day and invited you to work out with me at my corporate gym here in Houston. You jump in your car and stop at a service station to pick up a road map of Houston. When you finally get to Houston, you take the map out of your glove compartment. On the map, you locate the street and begin driving. Except that you notice right away that something isn't quite right. The street names you're passing don't match those on your map. You can't find the gym. Upon looking more closely at the map, you realize that what you have is actually a map of *Austin*, not Houston.

Now let's contemplate an alternate situation. Let's say that you never realize you have the wrong map. You drive around in circles, lost, but you're too proud (or bullheaded!) to call me for directions, so you "wing it." After driving around town for several hours, you give up in frustration.

The fact is, if you don't have the right map or directions, you fail to reach your destination. And you lose the motivation to keep going. While I'm waiting for you to show up, I have a great workout, drink a protein shake, and wonder where you are.

You can apply the same analogy to the majority of get-in-shape programs. If you start out with the wrong information, you are doomed to fail from the start.

There are many exercise and diet books on the market, each touting its own program of getting you into shape. There are dozens of TV infomercials touting exercise gadgets and pills, each promising you miracles. A trusting, uninitiated person looking for solutions can become confused with conflicting and oftentimes harmful information. To make matters worse, most people who try these misguided programs fail, and often then blame themselves for the failure. The result is frustration, unhappiness, and even guilt.

Reason #2: You Can't Sustain the Motivation

But it's not enough to be informed. Even if you have the right road map, you can never get to your destination if you don't take action and sustain action until you get there. Some people have the right road map, so to speak, but cannot get themselves motivated. Like a car that runs out of fuel, these people literally run out of willpower to continue their programs.

Motivation is the willpower to take action and sustain action on the information that you have. Motivation is to your efforts what fuel is to a car. When it comes to getting in shape, information plus motivation results in transformation, which is positive physical and mental change—the results that you want. Transformation is your destination. Look at it as the Lean Body Success Equation:

The Lean Body Success Equation:
Information (The Map) + *Motivation*
(The Fuel) = *Transformation*
(The Destination)

The Good News, the Bad News, and the Best News

I've talked about the importance of starting out with the right information. I've also talked about the importance of getting and staying motivated.

The good news is that I can give you the right road map. I know it's right because I have trained literally thousands of people who have used my Banex principle to get into and stay in the best shape of their lives.

The bad news is that I can't motivate you. *You* have to motivate you.

The best news is that if you give me an opportunity to help you, I can teach you to motivate yourself and stay motivated, and help you release the personal power that you have inside you. Motivation can be learned, and if applied correctly, it can become a life-long habit that can result in success in all areas of your life.

And What About Houston?

If you have any lingering doubts about the power of individuals to decide to change their bodies and their lives, let me introduce you to some friends of mine.

Namely, the citizens of Houston.

I can't tell you how proud I am of my hometown. In just one year, they managed to lose fat, build muscle, adopt healthier lifestyles, and make a promise to themselves to stay that way for as long as possible. In early January 2004, I was proud to appear on *Today* with the mayor of Houston to announce the news. Houston was no longer number one on the *Men's Fitness* Fattest Cities list.

America's Fattest Cities, 2004
(AS PER *MEN'S FITNESS* MAGAZINE)

1. Detroit, MI
2. **HOUSTON, TX**
3. Dallas, TX
4. San Antonio, TX
5. Chicago, IL

I helped to get Houston into shape and shed its title "America's Fattest City," just as I helped hundreds of thousands of people online. Now I'm extending my attention to the rest of the country and beyond. This is why I've written this book. I want to help you realize that getting in shape and staying in shape for the rest of your life can be as simple as turning the page.

Let's meet some other people who have overcome challenges to make the Lean Body Promise work for them.

They triumphed, and so can you.

PART TWO

The Inspiration

Americans love challenges. Give us a challenge, dare us to do something different, and we'll stun you with how hard we work to achieve our goals.

That's part of the reason why I created the Lean Body Challenge. In this part, you'll meet people who took the Challenge and found their inner lean body in just 12 weeks. They're not superheroes or genetic marvels. They're ordinary people. Some even had great odds to surmount, such as surprise surgery, adverse medical diagnoses, or accidents. Some simply had hectic schedules.

The Challenge was the direct offspring of the *Lean Body Coaching Club*. As I mentioned in the first part, this is a free weekly e-newsletter jam-packed with training tips and motivational articles on how to exercise, eat right, and achieve a leaner body.

Many of those members wanted to get back in shape but didn't know where to start. So I had the idea to give them a "virtual forum" in which to compete. A forum in which they would compete against themselves, and strut their stuff, so to speak, from the comfort of their own homes. Thus, the Lean Body Challenge.

The Lean Body Challenge was the first online-only competition of its kind, and we had a stunning response—so good that in the following year, we decided to present the Challenge again, not once but twice. All entrants were given a rigorous 12-week program, which is an abbreviated version of the Lean Body Promise. Taking the Challenge isn't easy, but the basic requirements are: simply snap a "before" photo and take your body measurements; follow the program to the best of your ability; then, finally, take some "after" photos and write an essay detailing how it all turned out.

Here are their stories.

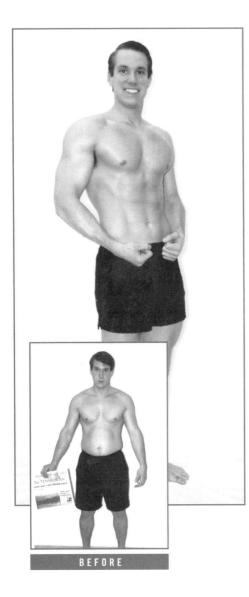

BEFORE

"She was everything."

Andrew Freck, Nashville, Tennessee

"Without Andy, I wouldn't have finished."

Paulina Soria, Antioch, Tennessee

Andrew Freck and Paulina Soria were a happy couple, but they weren't exactly happy with the way they looked. This changed when Paulina saw a reference to the Lean Body program. Even though their offices at their electrical supply company were just down the hall from each other, Paulina zapped Andrew an e-mail describing the program with the question: "Do you want to do this?"

Andrew thought about it. "To my surprise, I said yeah, let's do it."

Paulina was thrilled. But she assumed only one of them would be doing the Challenge.

"I have a condition called fibromyalgia, which makes weight-lifting difficult," says Paulina. Fibromyalgia is a muscle, ligament, and tendon disorder. (Imagine how your body feels when you have a bad case of the flu—achy and sore—then imagine feeling that way on a regular basis.) "I thought there was no way I could do this, but Andrew might be interested."

Andrew persisted. "Of course you can."

That's what did it for Paulina: Andrew's confidence in her. "Honestly, I didn't think I'd stick with it. But whenever I thought I couldn't do any more, Andrew would encourage me,

ANDREW'S LEAN BODY STATS

Pre-Challenge body fat index:	18%
Post-Challenge body fat index:	8%
NUMBER OF POUNDS LOST:	**22**

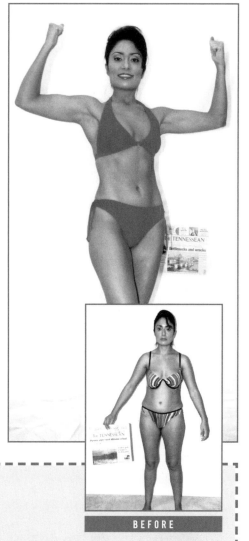

BEFORE

saying I could do it, I could quit if it started hurting." Eventually, Paulina could go for longer periods without pain, and her fibromyalgia symptoms seemed to ease up.

Soon after, Andrew and Paulina took their "before" photographs and got busy changing their lives. For starters, they planned a focused workout every day at lunchtime. Eventually, they even added a stationary bike routine before work. Once at work, the couple acted as each other's "food cops." Andrew would wander over to Paulina's office to make sure she was eating. Sometimes, it'd be Paulina making the run.

They did it . . . so can you!

Andrew and Paulina's Tips for Lean Body Success

1. Don't get discouraged. "The first weeks you go to the gym, if you can't do the exercises, don't get discouraged," says Paulina. "If you keep going and give it time, in three to four weeks you will be able to get through it. Just give your body time to adjust to a new routine and you can do it."

2. Consistency is key. "Consistency in performance, consistency in training—it's key to your results and the key to success in anything in life," says Andrew.

During the first two weeks, both Andrew and Paulina were surprised how much energy they had throughout the day. "In the past, I used to feel very tired around my lunchtime workouts," remembers Andrew. "For the second half of my day, I would never have much energy to do anything else—not even work." But on the Lean Body program, both felt like they were fully alert and vibrant throughout the day, from dawn to dusk.

From there, the changes seemed to appear fast and furious. From there, the changes seemed to appear fast and furious. "They came from nowhere!" says Paulina. "You'll be like, where did I get that muscle from? It's an incredible confirmation. The last month of the program was especially revealing. After enough body fat had burned up, I started seeing muscles I'd never seen before!"

"It's amazing how just ten pounds can make a difference in your physique and appearance," says Andrew.

Twelve weeks seemed to fly, and when Andrew and Paulina went to take their "after" photos, they were surprised. "I never thought I could look like that," says Paulina. "My sister is the one who took my 'before' picture. When she finished taking the 'after' picture, she said, 'Oh my God—whatever you did to get that body, I want to do it, too.'" Note: This is the same twin sister who, throughout their entire lives, seemed just a bit thinner and more in shape than Paulina. "I was so proud," she says.

"If Andy wasn't there to help me through the rough times, I don't think I would have finished," says Paulina.

"Same for me," says Andrew. "To have a coach, a friend, a workout partner, and a diet partner through all this—she was everything."

"There's always a way."

Kevin Saunders, Downs, Kansas

In early April 1981, Kevin Saunders had a degree from Kansas State University, a new job in South Texas, and a beautiful wife who was pregnant with their son. Kevin was working on a grain elevator on a farm in Corpus Christi when there was a sudden explosion. The blast ripped through 2 feet of reinforced concrete and killed 10 men instantly. It also sent Kevin hurling over 300 feet through the air before his body slammed into a concrete parking lot. His lungs collapsed. His spinal cord was shattered.

But Kevin refused to give up. "After my injury, I didn't know if I wanted to live. I'd been married nine months and two days, and my wife gave birth to our boy while I was still in the hospital. But then I started to pray for strength, and I knew I had to have some purpose on the earth."

Once the stunned doctors realized he was going to survive the accident, Kevin became determined to become a wheelchair athlete. Now he just had to learn to utilize the functional parts of his body; the accident had left him paralyzed from the waist down. "I learned at that early age that being in shape was critical if I wanted to travel the world. So I had to depend on my arms to take me places."

That single-minded determination turned Kevin into one of the most successful

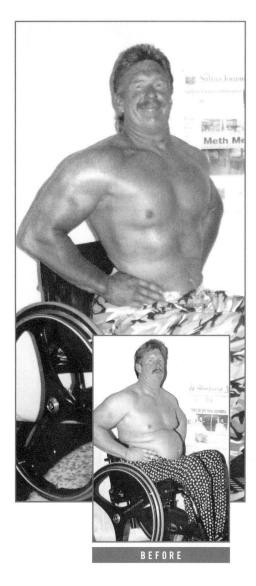

BEFORE

KEVIN'S LEAN BODY STATS

Pre-Challenge body fat index:	29.4%
Post-Challenge body fat index:	12.7%
NUMBER OF POUNDS LOST:	**40**

disabled athletes during the 1980s, scooping up gold medals by the handful, appearing in the Oliver Stone movie *Born on the Fourth of July*, and being named by President George H. W. Bush to the President's Council on Physical Fitness and Sports.

Then a little over 20 years after the Corpus Christi explosion that changed Kevin's life, fate came calling again.

"I had an accident," says Kevin. "Yeah, another one, if you can believe it. During my six months of bed rest, I overate and got completely out of shape. My waist ballooned to 48 inches, and it's usually 34." It was another blow in a life that already absorbed a massive blow.

Still, he decided to reclaim the body he'd once had. And to do it, he chose the Lean Body program. "Was it tough? I'm not going to say it was easy. But you have to remember this isn't a quick fix. It's a lifestyle change."

Kevin has toured 148 cities across the country, spreading the idea that if he can transform his body, anybody else can, too.

"I wanted to be an inspiration to my clients."

Darrell Collins, Plattsburgh, New York

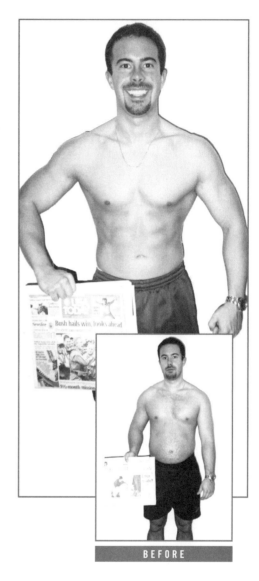

I n Darrell Collins's part of the country—upstate New York—health and fitness are not exactly an obsession. After all, this is the state where they invented Buffalo wings.

In college, Darrell became serious about nutrition. His goal was to become a personal trainer and nutritional advisor upon graduation from Plattsburgh State University. As anyone with a bachelor's degree can attest, the collegiate lifestyle is usually full of late-night pizza, keg parties, odd nutrition habits (the same late-night pizza, cold, for breakfast), and a host of skipped workouts in favor of taking naps. The result for Darrell? His worst physical shape ever.

When Darrell was a senior, he got a job as the assistant manager at the local fitness facility, advising clients on nutrition guidelines and workout routines.

Darrell, 22, knew that to sound credible, he had to look authoritative. That's when he found the Labrada website. Once Darrell saw the Lean Body Challenge, he knew it was something he had to try.

For Darrell, the tough part wasn't schlepping to the gym. And it wasn't necessarily the meal plan. It was his hectic schedule—9:30 A.M. college classes, papers, reading assign-

DARRELL'S LEAN BODY STATS	
Pre-Challenge body fat index:	20%
Post-Challenge body fat index:	6%
NUMBER OF POUNDS LOST:	**30**

He did it . . . so can you!

Darrell's Tips for Lean Body Success

1. **Take it one day at a time.** Daily affirmations—yeah, I can do this!—will fuel your motivation and help you go the distance.

2. **Don't panic.** Darrell always kept a practical outlook on occasional eating slipups: he refused to let them throw him off course. "One meal isn't going to ruin you. Just hop back on the horse as soon as possible and keep riding."

ments, and well-meaning friends who want to drag you off to a sports pub for pizza and pitchers. Darrell pushed on anyway.

Soon enough, the semester—and the Challenge—drew to a close, and a brand-new Darrell Collins emerged. He had earned his B.S. in food and nutrition . . . and lost 30 pounds. "Finally, I felt like I looked the part," he said. Now that he's lean, Darrell says he finds it easier to be a "fitness evangelist," spreading the good word to the clients he guides every day at the gym.

Since Darrell has become quite professional at motivating people, I thought I'd let him have the last word on why you should consider taking the Lean Body Challenge yourself.

"What you've accomplished with your body is better than any kind of prize," he says. "And looking back, it really wasn't that hard."

"I'm tired of carrying the extra baggage."

Earl Bailey, Canton, Ohio

I n the 1970s, Earl Bailey's life was a nice balance of the physical and the spiritual. "I was the pastor of a good-sized, growing church, and I was very involved in the local high school football program as chaplain and coach," says Bailey, a robust athlete. "Then I was diagnosed with multiple sclerosis in 1978. I was told that I would most likely lose my ability to walk." Earl was only 38.

At first, Earl was determined to outrun the MS. "I continued to exercise, pushing myself to go beyond what I had ever done. For a while, I stayed fairly well." Earl even entered and won third place in a "Hall of Fame" body-building tournament two years after the diagnosis. "But then my legs started to go." First came the cane. Then a set of forearm crutches. Finally, even those devices failed to help Earl walk unassisted. "I ended up on an electric cart."

Still, Earl never thought about quitting his workout routine completely. Time and again he'd be forced to stop after a few months of working out due to the excruciating pain. Even a spinal cord stimulator failed to diminish the pain. Finally, he called it quits, but that hurt even worse than the pain of the MS.

Several months later, Earl's youngest son became curious about weight lifting and asked his father to work out with him. This coin-

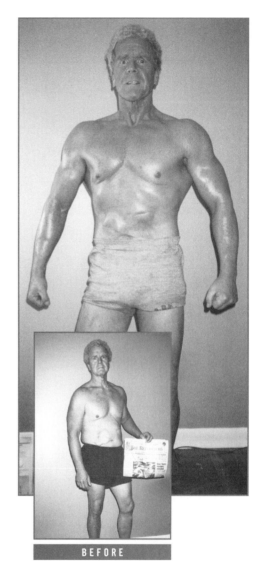

BEFORE

EARL'S LEAN BODY STATS	
Pre-Challenge body fat index:	18%
Post-Challenge body fat index:	9%
NUMBER OF POUNDS LOST:	**21**

The Inspiration   **25**

cided with Earl hearing about the Lean Body Challenge. "The contest gave me just the right boost to say, 'This is it! I'm tired of carrying the extra baggage and looking like I do.'"

By this time, Earl had managed to forgo the wheelchair. But then came a surprise abdominal surgery—another in a long series of surgeries that has plagued Earl since 1978—not long before the competition began. The pain was so great, doctors had implanted a pump that injected a steady flow of morphine directly into his spine. Earl recovered in time to begin the workouts and nutrition routine, but it wasn't easy. He was starting from scratch.

Despite the pain, Earl completed 20 to 30 minutes of cardio work five days a week, followed by my weight training program. Not even two trips to the hospital threw him completely off course. By the end of the Challenge, Earl had lost 22 pounds, dropped five full pant sizes, and started fooling people who didn't believe he could possibly be in his sixties. Earl didn't win the Challenge, but not one to give up, he decided to enter the Challenge again.

That's right; Earl had decided to enter the Challenge again. "This time my goal was to still lose fat but *not* body weight."

The second time around, Earl ended up capturing first place in his age division, as well as the "most inspirational" award. To me, Earl is the perfect example of how anyone, at any age, can overcome life's most challenging hurdles and end up even stronger and happier than before.

He did it . . . so can you!

Earl's Tips for Lean Body Success

1. Believe you can. "Someone—many have taken credit for this quote—said, 'If you believe you can or believe you can't, you're absolutely right,'" says Earl.

2. Take joy in the physical results. "No matter what your age, it always feels good to be able to take your shirt off and not see your belly hanging over your belt."

Listen to This

Being surrounded by delicious, high-calorie foods and not allocating time for exercise had gradually transformed me into the stereotypical roly-poly pizza man. Before the Lean Body Challenge, I really wasn't active at all—well, besides tossing pizzas. To be honest, it was hard to get started. I didn't realize how much weight I'd gained until I took the "before" picture.

It didn't take long to realize that by eating healthy and exercising, I was dramatically improving my overall quality of life. I feel better and my attitude each day is positive and energetic. I demand more of myself and I fulfill my promises. I absolutely love the changes I've made in my life.

Dave Dunham is the co-owner of a pizzeria in Staten Island, New York.

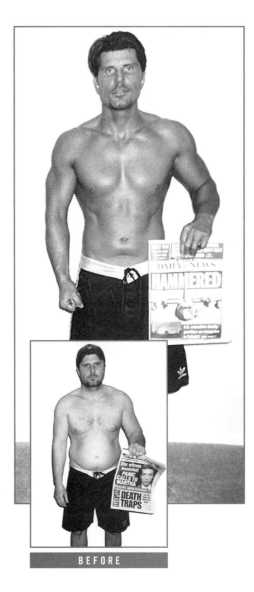

BEFORE

"I wanted a six-pack and now I have it."

George Tardibono, Oklahoma City, Oklahoma

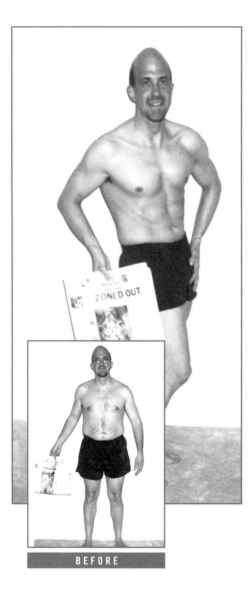

BEFORE

t's no secret that America is in the throes of an obesity epidemic. And doctors are the workers on the front lines, performing triage on their patients with nutrition and fitness advice. But what happens when doctors themselves fall prey to the epidemic?

Dr. George Tardibono was one of those medical doctors. He wasn't obese, certainly; he just wasn't completely satisfied with his physique—not his 34-inch pant size, or his 159-pound frame. "As a physician, I hear a myriad of complaints from patients as to why they can't lose weight," says Dr. Tardibono. "I thought that I would enter the Challenge to have some proof to tell them that it *can* be done. As someone they can see personally, this might spur them on to better health as well."

The Lean Body Challenge helps people to be accountable. "I wanted to see if I could change my body composition significantly as compared to my twin brother, who was not going to be in the Challenge," admits Dr. Tardibono. "He served—unknowingly—as the control subject."

The first weeks of the Challenge were full of simple treadmill routines—20 minutes per day, four days a week, which he eventually expanded to 45 minutes per session. Dr. Tardibono's weight routine was simple, too: 45 minutes to an hour of weight lifting using the most basic of home gym equipment: dumbbells, a lift bar, and a bench.

Two months flew by, and Dr. Tardibono started to see the results he'd been after. But then came a speed bump in the third month: a month of making rounds with medical students, which can be one of the most intense work periods in a doctor's life. His workload increased, his workouts suffered, and it was tough to squeeze in every meal. But he refused to give up. Dr. Tardibono simply made adjustments to fit his harried schedule. If he couldn't eat a complete Lean Body meal, he made a point of snacking on something healthy—even just a granola bar—instead of something out of a hospital vending machine.

By the Challenge's end, and despite the time constraints, Dr. Tardibono had stunningly achieved his goal: a leaner body that could serve as an example to his patients. He had vaporized 15 pounds of fat and dropped down two full pant sizes. Oh, and of course, there was that *other* goal. The one he could see whenever he lifted up his shirt. "I wanted a six-pack, and now I have it!" says Dr. Tardibono.

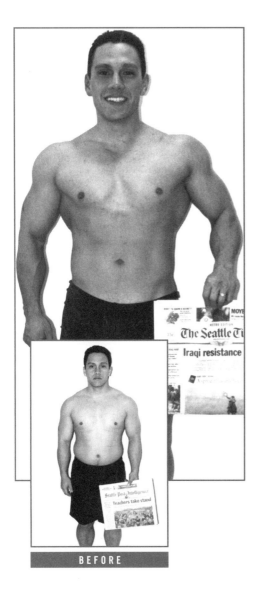

BEFORE

Listen to This

I teach in an elementary school, so I thought it was important to set a healthy example for my students. Nutrition is not discussed enough in the classroom—some kids actually think a candy bar is a healthy snack. After a few weeks on the Lean Body program, I started becoming leaner and more muscular, and my students started taking notice. They asked a million questions, and they really got interested when I started explaining how goal setting helped me to achieve a lean, stronger body. Suddenly, the idea of a healthy lifestyle became real—and important—to them. I wanted to try and do something that is manageable in the long term, and all the things I've done with this program I can maintain throughout my life.

Joe Malek is an elementary school teacher in Seattle, Washington.

"It's a really great feeling!"

Carrie Shipp, Dallas, Texas

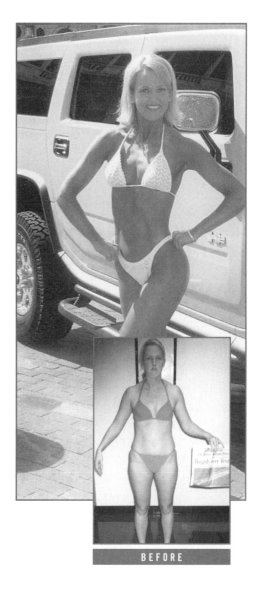

BEFORE

Carrie Shipp wants to get one thing straight: she wasn't a slouch when it came to health and fitness. The hardworking airline employee used to have a hard time with healthy eating. "I yo-yo dieted quite a bit, but never achieved the shape I wanted," she explains. One day, she decided, *Enough already.* Carrie started a regimen of healthy eating habits and visits to the gym and managed to drop four dress sizes over a period of two years.

Carrie's goal was to build the best body possible—and specifically, drop a few more dress sizes. "This goal positively lit a fire inside me," she says. "It kept me strong when I felt tired." It also helped that Carrie kept not only her goal in mind, but the path to the goal as well. "I planned and rehearsed my success in my head so that giving up never entered my mind. It became routine, just what I did every day." Visualization is a powerful tool; if you can imagine yourself doing something, your brain eventually responds. Soon, you *will* be able to do it.

As for workouts, Carrie used my program as her guideline. She exercised nearly every day, incorporating weight training and cardio. What was Carrie packing for lunch and snacks? "I ate lots of egg whites, chicken, vegetables, and oatmeal," she says, "plus the occasional snack or free meal."

CARRIE'S LEAN BODY STATS

Pre-Challenge body fat index:	22%
Post-Challenge body fat index:	12.8%
NUMBER OF POUNDS LOST:	**18**

She did it . . . so can you!

Carrie's Tips for Lean Body Success

1. **Having a bad day? Don't give up.** "Just continue stringing the days together and doing the best you can," says Carrie. "No one does everything perfectly. The mountain called fitness isn't as hard to climb as people think. It's just an accumulation of baby steps until you reach the top."

2. **Doing it is easier than not doing it.** "I believe it's far easier to do what needs to be done for the day—working out, eating right—than fretting about missing a day," says Carrie. "You can spend all day beating yourself up over the fact that you missed a day of training. Or you can simply take the hour or so necessary to do it and feel great about yourself all day."

3. **Remember: this will all pay off in the end.** "Follow every instruction, take the pictures and measurements," says Carrie. This is an incredibly important step. It will reinforce your commitment and fuel your motivation. "You will love looking back at your accomplishment. Commit to the program fully and watch the butterfly within you emerge."

The most important thing: it worked for her. Big time. Carrie cut her body fat percentage nearly in half, lost close to 20 pounds, and went from a size 8 dress to a size 2. I'm also proud to say that Carrie won the title of Grand Champion during a recent Lean Body Challenge. But for our champ, this is just the beginning.

"When you take care of your body and fuel it properly, you are able to unleash your best self," Carrie says. "Now I'm pursuing things in my life that had previously intimidated me. People turn to me for training advice and motivation. It's a really great feeling to help others and give them hope."

"Now this is how I want to look and feel."

Michael Camelo, Cape Coral, Florida

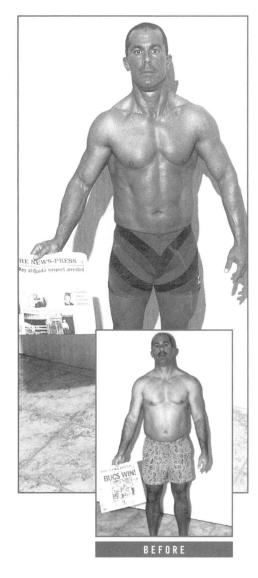

BEFORE

W ant to know how to insult another firefighter? Brown-bag your dinner.

"Firefighters are known as great cooks," explains Michael Camelo, a 46-year-old fireman in Cape Coral, Florida. Everyone kicks in some money to pay for lunch and dinner, and the most talented cooks in the house whip up the menu based on the size of the budget. "So brown-bagging is frowned upon."

That presented a small dilemma for Michael, who had realized that he was unhappy with his physical condition. Obviously, firefighters need to be in top physical condition to withstand the rigors of battling blazes and rescuing their fellow citizens (as well as the occasional feline). But for Michael, it was a bit more personal. He'd been an active athlete and recreational weight lifter for most of his life, but as he approached his forties, his activity had slowed down considerably. The inactivity was taking a physical toll.

Also, Michael had recently been named the head of the Health and Safety Committee at his department, which means he was basically the fitness "watchdog" in his house. Michael knew he needed something to motivate him; he found it in the Lean Body Challenge.

Since the life of a firefighter can be calm one minute and chaotic the next, Michael de-

MICHAEL'S LEAN BODY STATS	
Pre-Challenge body fat index:	26%
Post-Challenge body fat index:	11%
NUMBER OF POUNDS LOST:	15

The Inspiration 33

cided to ensure he always had the opportunity to work out. "There was stuff at the firehouse, but I also bought equipment for home—I just didn't have time to go back and forth to a gym." No matter where he was, Michael did cardio daily.

But what about the times when the alarm bells started ringing? "If I had to go on a call, I could always throw the thermos on the truck. Don't get me wrong—I wouldn't let it interfere with fighting fires. But after the action had settled down, I'd have my next meal ready to go."

And Michael even found a solution for the brown-bagging dilemma. "I decided to bring my Lean Body meals with me, but I still paid in," says Michael.

Michael's colleagues were extremely supportive—and eventually envious. Over the course of just 12 weeks, Michael had lost 15 pounds and dropped two full pant sizes. "When I came back and told them where I'd placed in the Challenge, they couldn't believe it. In fact, after Christmas, some of the guys said, 'I gotta get on that diet you were on.'"

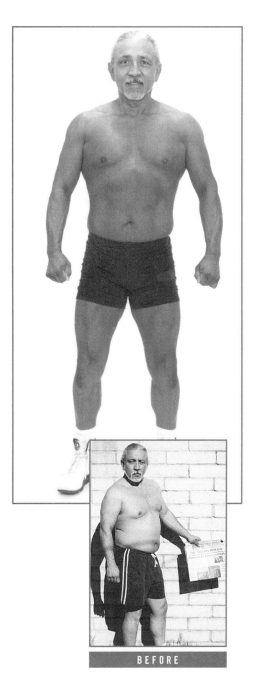

BEFORE

Listen to This

My overall goal was to lose the weight. I reached that goal, and I'm doing pretty well at maintaining it. I knew I'd made a difference when I saw the expression on other people's faces. Even better is the fact that I can help others do the same thing. I volunteer every Sunday and teach a kickboxing class at the YMCA. Losing the weight really helped me to motivate other people to actually try to reach their goals. Plus, I feel so energized that making those kicks is a breeze!

Frank Aquirre is a native of Phoenix, Arizona.

Now that you've met some of the ordinary people who have made extraordinary changes in their lives . . . are you ready to follow in their footsteps? You should have no doubt in your mind that no matter your life situation, you are in control and empowered to make long-lasting changes in your body. Now it's time for the next step: getting you motivated. It's going to be easier than you think.

In fact, all you have to do is turn to the next chapter.

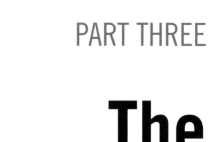

PART THREE

The Motivation

I'm going to hand you the five foolproof keys to motivating yourself, anytime, anywhere. There are no batteries, tapes, or gadgets required. In fact, the only materials you need to successfully change your entire outlook on health and fitness are in the book you're holding in your hands, plus a pen, some index cards, and a wall calendar. That's it.

You should know up front that there is no instant motivation "pill." In fact, that's the hidden lie behind many fitness gimmicks and nutrition fads: they claim that their program is so short and so easy, you don't need an ounce of motivation. Sadly, that quick-fix mentality—*I'm just going to get through this once, and I'll never have to do it again*—will only lead you right back to where you started. And you'll be $39.95 (or $79.95, or $295.95) poorer for the experience.

I want to help you develop a nutrition and exercise program that you can live with on a day-to-day basis and that doesn't make you miserable. You won't have to "put up" with the Lean Body program; you'll enjoy living it and you'll enjoy the daily rewards you receive from it. You can win the battle for the body you desire on a day-by-day basis. The more you make the right choices—to eat right and exercise—the easier it will become over time.

That's right: it will become easier over time, guaranteed. First we have to understand the forces that tie us to our old, negative habits.

Overcoming the Ties That Bind

Imagine you're standing in a room between two walls. You're facing a wall that we're going to call "desired outcome." Maybe that wall has an image of you at 20 pounds lighter and three dress or pant sizes smaller. A healthier, happier, leaner you. You very much want to reach that wall. The wall behind you? That's called "the way things are."

What do you do to reach the desired outcome? You walk toward it. But wait; there's a catch. Seems there's a large elastic band around your waist tethering you to the wall behind you. Every time you step toward your desired outcome, the band stretches and the tension increases, trying to pull you back to the way things are. You want to reach that desired outcome so badly, but that blasted band is getting tighter and tighter and tighter. . . .

Anytime you try to break out of an old habit, there's a certain amount of negative tension that tries to pull you back toward that old habit. That's because your mind is like a cranky grandfather: it has an internal resistance to change. It's simply more comfortable to have things pegged. That wall behind you? It's familiar turf. Safe. Understandable.

The wall behind you is made of a number of routines we call habits. Good or bad, these habits become hardwired into our psyche by rote, and it's uncomfortable to break out of them. To change our habits, we have to consciously work hard at it. Even when we succeed, we then have to make sure we replace them with something else—good habits.

The lesson here is that when you have a desired outcome and work toward it, you're going to initially have internal resistance. If you keep at it, however, you will eventually reach the point where your positive actions will overpower the negative tension. The rubber band will snap, and you'll go flying toward your desired outcome. Hopefully not too hard.

That's what motivation boils down to: countering the negative tension that tries to pull you back with positive action to propel you forward. This chapter will teach you some ways to loosen the strangling hold of that rubber band.

THE SKINNY SO FAR . . .

▌ There's no such thing as a "quick fix" to a healthy lifestyle. But the good news? The more you work at it, the easier it gets over time.

▌ Tension sounds bad—but it can be a good thing, once you learn how to harness its power.

▌ If you hang in there long enough, you'll reach a point where you overcome the negative tension and you'll reach your goals more quickly.

So What's Holding You Back?

Typically, there are three things tying us back to our old habits: fear, excuses, and negative self-talk.

#1. Fear Itself

A certain amount of fear is good. Are you afraid of running across a busy interstate at rush hour? That's a healthy fear. Afraid of stepping too close to the edge of a tall building while blindfolded? Another healthy fear. If human beings weren't hardwired with a certain amount of fear, we wouldn't have made it out of prehistoric times alive.

Many fears, however, are unfounded in reality. And these fears are the ones that stop you from trying. "I failed before," you might say. "Why should I do this to myself again?" Once your fears are reinforced, you might ask, "Why should I bother in the first place?"

Thing is, you do have a choice. You need to think about what's holding you back instead of being dominated by fear. Here's an acronym I call to mind when I start seeing shadows on the wall:

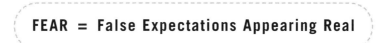

FEAR = False Expectations Appearing Real

And most times, that's all that you're afraid of: false expectations. *I'll never finish it. It won't work on me. I'll screw it up.* These are all not true. They're phantoms, easily dispelled with a little positive thinking. But getting trapped in a perpetual downward spiral of negative thinking will lock up your ability to think through a problem and come up with a breakthrough solution. Fear will hold back the very thing that can help.

Your desire to reach the outcome—a leaner, healthier body—must be stronger than the fear that keeps you back. There's going to be a certain amount of discomfort in approaching any goal. Your desire has to be stronger. If you can make that desire real enough—crystallize it in your mind—you'll be able to outpace your fear.

#2. Excuses, Excuses

Want to know the difference between achievers and nonachievers? It's in the way they face negative situations in their lives. Nonachievers use their situation as an excuse to give up; achievers use their situation as a reason to change.

On the surface, the excuses might sound perfectly reasonable—"I'm simply too fat"; "I've done this before"; "I don't have time to eat right or work out"—but they're unfounded roadblocks to success. Most excuse-makers find themselves waiting for something in the universe to change before they do, such as: "I'll lose five pounds, then I'll go to the gym." That's an excuse. Why not start right now?

Motivation Tip #1

An excuse is a psychological crutch. It allows you a comfortable way to postpone an action that you know you should really take today. When you take action immediately, you always feel better about yourself afterward.

#3. Negative Self-Talk

There are voices inside my head. They're inside yours, too.

Don't call a psychiatrist just yet. Everybody has voices inside their heads. I'm referring to the mental chatter we all have going on—What should I have for lunch today . . . hmmm, that peach looks nice . . . whoah, piece of lint on my pants . . . there we go . . . into the trash . . . what was I thinking? . . . oh yeah, lunch . . . —all the time, 24/7. This mental chatter can be positive or negative.

Unfortunately, negative chatter is the default position for most people, unless they're careful to monitor their internal dialogue. Some of us beat ourselves up—*I'm no good at this* or *I can't do anything right*—which sometimes echoes someone in the past, such as a schoolteacher or hypercritical adult. You say it enough times, and you start to believe it. Motivation breaks down when you entertain negative self-talk.

It's not unlike programming a computer—what's the Silicon Valley saying? Garbage in, garbage out. But this isn't a modern concept. One of my favorite motivational writers, James Allen, wrote about the same idea back in the 1800s in *As a Man Thinketh*. Allen describes the mind as a garden. You can plant positive seeds (thoughts) in the fertile soil and receive positive results, or you can plant negative seeds in the soil that yield nothing but negative results. Or you can plant nothing at all, in which case you'll have a garden full of weeds.

Self-talk may be defeating you. Whenever a negative thought pops into your head, you need to replace it with a positive one. Even if it seems like a futile effort at first, stay at it. Eventually it will get easier.

Breaking Free of Bad Habits

How long does it take to break or change a bad habit? From my personal experience, I know that it takes about a month to establish a new habit. If you can stick with my program through the first month, it'll likely become habit for you.

What I'm asking for is not a test of your endurance—something that you'll want to end as soon as possible. I'm asking you to look at your life in a different way—a paradigm shift. Instead of looking at workouts and a smart nutrition plan as temporary drudgery to endure for 12 weeks, look at it as a personal investment.

Let's say that in the past you tried to get into shape, but fell into the habit of blowing off your workouts from time to time. This can lead to stagnation in your routine, or eventually, you opting to not renew your gym membership. How do you improve the situation? Make a commitment to work out first thing in the morning, no matter how tired you feel. Commit to this for just one month.

During the first week, this will be very tough. You're not going to like yourself in the mornings. You'll probably need to give yourself pep talks.

By week two, it'll still be tough. Sorry.

But by weeks three and four, you'll notice that it starts becoming easier and natural to work out first thing in the morning. It will start to become part of your "internal self"—Yep, that's me, Mr./Ms. Workout-Every-Morning.

Once you start telling yourself that, you've successfully replaced the negative habit (skipping workouts) with a positive one (getting your workouts done every day). In fact, you'll notice a 180-degree shift. Once you're working out regularly, you'll actually feel depressed if you a *skip* a workout. Your body has become used to that daily release of mood-elevating endorphins (feel-good brain chemicals). This negative feeling can actually reinforce your new positive habit.

Consistency is the key to changing a negative habit. You must make the commitment to do something about your shape and your physical condition each and every day, day after day, week after week, month after month. Many people start fitness or diet programs and quit after a few days or weeks. A period of time elapses, and they lose the results they gained during their initial burst of enthusiasm, and they embark on yet another fitness or diet program. This series of starts and stops stalls their progress. On the other hand, if you were to make an investment in yourself every day, just imagine the results you would have.

Now that you recognize what you're up against—your fears, excuses, and negative self-talk—let's talk about the five specific ways you can beat the odds and reach your desired outcome.

THE SKINNY SO FAR . . .

▌ Fear, excuses, and negative self-talk are the three most common forces that hold you back from your goals.

▌ Once you replace a negative habit with a positive one, that positive habit will become part of your "internal self."

▌ Consistency is the key. If you can keep up the program for even just a few weeks, you'll reinforce your positive habits, making it much easier to stick with it.

Step #1: Set Realistic Goals

Every voyage begins with a goal. It's much better if you have a *realistic* goal.

You might say to yourself: *Okay—I'm going to lose 20 pounds in two weeks and lose three belt sizes!* That's an ambitious goal. But unless you know what is physiologically possible, you'll be setting yourself up for failure. I wouldn't want you to set a goal that is next to impossible to achieve, or achieved in an unhealthy way. Fact is, if you lose more than two to three pounds per week, you end up burning muscle tissue and slowing your metabolism. Plus, you'll feel deprived and even more tempted to binge.

Motivation Tip #2

It always helps to give yourself a solid timeline to achieve results. When you hold yourself accountable to a fixed timeline, you summon a sense of purpose and commitment to your pursuit.

You can safely lose about two to three pounds of fat per week without hitting a starvation mode or losing muscle. So over 12 weeks, you can reasonably expect 15 to 35 pounds of fat to drop off. How much depends on how well you eat and exercise. It wouldn't surprise me if, over the course of the Lean Body program, you added 10 pounds of lean muscle while simultaneously dropping 20 pounds of body fat. As we'll soon find out, lean muscle is a good thing, giving your body shape in the right places.

Get Out Your Pen! (Part I) ✎

Surveys have shown that only a small percentage of people actually write down their life goals. The vast majority of people are just "winging it."

It's critically important to write down a goal and put it on a timeline. Goal-setting gives you a clearly defined objective to build a routine around. Plus, writing it down makes it real. We have thousands of thoughts going through our heads every day. But when we write something down and put it in a place where we can see it, we've taken the first step toward assimilating it. Don't be timid or afraid to set those goals. Put them on paper.

I mean it. Right now. Here in this book. (If you don't want to write in your book, photocopy this page or use two index cards.)

Write down your goals—for the 12-week program, then for the coming year. What would you like to accomplish?

MY 12-WEEK GOAL:

THE LEAN BODY *PROMISE*

One sample goal: "I want to drop 20 pounds of fat, add five pounds of lean muscle tissue, take two inches off my waist, and add a half inch to my arms or legs."

MY 12-MONTH GOAL:

One sample goal: "I want to lose 40 pounds of fat, drop my body fat percentage by 15 points, and achieve that six-pack I've always wanted."

Thanks for taking this first step. It's more important than you might think. Now let's move on to the next motivational key.

Step #2: Take Back Control of Your Mind

Did you ever listen to a song—even a song you hate—and then suddenly you can't get it out of your head? It's amazing how the brain sponges up information. You think: *Boy, I hate this song. I really, really hate this song. I wish they'd stop playing this song.* Your brain absorbs: *Song. Song. Song.* All of a sudden, it's going through your head all the time. Which is really awful if the song happens to be "Afternoon Delight."

The lesson: Never underestimate the power of suggestion—or your mind, for that matter. This is why it's important to weed out those negative, self-defeating thoughts and replace them with positive, goal-achieving thoughts. Instead of saying, *I'm no good,* say, *I'm getting better every day.* When that negative thought flies back into your head, just push it out again. After a while, it becomes easier, more effortless. With time, you'll have fewer negative thoughts.

Positive self-affirmations are short strings of words that specifically describe your desired outcomes or goals. Your positive self-affirmation phrases become a mantra that you repeat to yourself at key times during the day. Through repetition, your subconscious mind assimilates and internalizes your goals. Your brain will be working on them even when you are not consciously thinking of them, and your self-affirmations will guide your every move toward your goals.

So how do you write and use a positive self-affirmation?

1. *Make sure your positive self-affirmations are . . . well, positive.* Instead of saying, *I will not eat junk foods,* say, *I will eat only lean foods.* The thing is, your brain doesn't recognize the word "not"; it hears "junk food." When you say, *I will not eat junk food,* your brain thinks, *Mmmmmm. Chips. Could go for some right about now.*

2. *Put it in terms of the present, as if you are already accomplishing it.* Otherwise, your brain will put the affirmation on its long-term "to-do list," which has been collecting dust in the back of your head somewhere since 1989. For example, say, *I am losing 10 pounds of fat,* instead of *I will lose 10 pounds of fat.*

3. *Commit to repeating your mantras for at least a month.* Again, this is the amount of time it takes to develop a habit. Don't give up if you don't start seeing results in 48 hours. It's like exercising only two times and saying, *Hey, my arms aren't growing. What the heck's going on here? I've been on this program two whole days!* Likewise, planting positive thoughts will take more than a few half-hearted repetitions.

Motivation Tip #3

Can you visualize the body you want to have? Then you've made an important first step toward *achieving* that body. Keep that picture in your head. The next step is to take sustained action in pursuit of your goal.

At first, you're going to be saying, "Gimme a break. This is hokey." That's normal. We live in an era of sarcasm and cynicism. But you don't need to repeat your self-affirmation out loud ten times, or bellow it in your best James Earl Jones impression. Just kick it around your head as much as possible.

Trust me: If you say the darn thing enough, I promise you, your mind is going to soak up the data and it's going to find a way to plant that in your subconscious. And then it will manifest itself physically.

Get Out Your Pen! (Part II) ✏️

You already have your goals written down. Now, on a separate index card, write a self-affirmation. Keep it nearby so you can access it every day.

MY SELF-AFFIRMATION:

Be specific. Don't write down something vague, like "I'm getting into shape." Instead write:

"I'm losing 10 pounds of fat. And I'm losing two inches from my waist."

Or:

"I'm losing 20 pounds of fat, and I'm going from a dress size 9 to a size 5."

Got something in mind? Good. Now make three copies and . . .

1. Keep one posted on the bathroom mirror.
2. Keep another posted on your bedside table.
3. Put the third in your purse or wallet, where you can refer to it.

Why these three places? People usually start their day in the bathroom. You wake up, look in the mirror, mutter, "You handsome devil," and brush your teeth. That's when you should reread that self-affirmation. It's important because at the very beginning of the day when you're coming out of sleep, you're in a twilight zone. At that time, your subconscious is very permeable to instruction and suggestion.

Dwell on that goal in the shower—what else are you going to do there? Read the *Wall Street Journal*? During the day, if you find yourself needing a boost, look at your self-affirmation. Then again at night, right before you drift off to golden slumbers, read it yet again. Your subconscious will work on the challenge you've given it, even while you're snoozing.

Step #3: Find a Body Buddy

Fun. That's the one thing missing from exercise these days. When we were kids, there was always a heavy element of play with sports. You may have been trying to annihilate little Jeffy with the dodgeball, but you were also running around like a maniac, working muscles and pumping blood and oxygen throughout your body. You were a lean, mean, dodgeball-hurling machine.

But now we're adults. And what do people think about when they think "exercise"? Resistance training, lifting weights, riding a bike. To some, those activities are not a lot of fun. Especially if you're doing it by yourself. So how can you make it more fun? Find a body buddy.

Ideally, you want someone who shares your enthusiasm, your goals, and may even sign up for the Lean Body program with you. Having a body buddy makes you accountable—you're less likely to miss a workout.

Secondly, your body buddy can help motivate you. No one is completely "up" every single day. There may be a day you don't feel like working out. But if you drag yourself to the gym anyway, your buddy can pick you up by the shorts and dust you off. Before you know it, you're a few sets into it, your blood is pumping, and you feel good again.

The ideal body buddy is someone who will show up on time and is motivating, not de-motivating. Choose someone who shares similar goals and is equal to you in condition and strength.

If you can't find or don't want a body buddy, I can help. You can count on me every week to provide free support at the Lean Body Coach website (www.leanbodycoach.com).

Step #4: Get Feedback

You've selected a realistic goal. You've regained control of your mind. You've even found a body buddy. What's the next step? *Enjoying* your new Lean Body Promise routine.

That's right; I used the word "enjoy." It's vital that you make the mental link between this program and "fun." If you're doing all of this hard work in a vacuum and not deriving any pleasure during those 12 weeks, it's going to be difficult for you to continue. You're going to approach this as just more diet and exercise drudgery, something to *live through* instead of to *live*.

So where's the fun? In the rewards, baby.

By "rewards" I mean the daily and weekly triumphs—not just your 12-week goal, one-year goal, or lifetime goal. I'm talking about enjoying the feeling of your body working and sweating. And finally, I mean the small changes in your body that can be measured and relished. This is what I call "feedback," and it's at the very heart of motivation.

Motivation Tip #4

There's nothing like your first hit of positive feedback to make you realize that you can achieve your goals. The trick to making a lifestyle change is setting up ways to receive steady, positive feedback. True, we can't win physique contests or bikini pageants every day. But seeing your body fat percentage slipping down a few digits at a time can be just as inspiring.

For your progress to be satisfying on an ongoing basis, it's important to measure it . . . repeatedly. And as a beginner, you have to allow yourself enough time to reach at least that first stage where you see the physical fruits of your labor. If you can hang in long enough to see the first wave of results, you'll most likely stick it out for the long haul. *My goodness*, you'll say to yourself. *I'm 5 pounds lighter!* That's the reward. Suddenly, you want to do it again.

Feedback can take many forms. The most obvious is your image in the mirror, but checking your progress this way can be tough, because changes tend to be gradual and hard to see.

A preferred form of feedback is physical measurements, which measure real progress. Here are five of the best ways:

1. *Measure body fat.* This method estimates how much of your body tissue is made up of fat. The measurement is especially useful because it can tell you when you're dropping body fat, as opposed to overall weight. You'll need a set of body fat calipers, but fortunately, I've made that inexpensive and easy for you. See Appendix D for a special offer to readers of this book, as well as a simple tutorial on how to use them.

It's important not to get hung up on the absolute measurement given by the body fat calipers: it's just an estimate. But, you'll want to pay attention to how that number changes from week to week. The relative change in numbers will be accurate, as long as the measurements are taken the same way each time.

2. *Hop on a scale.* We're all familiar with this time-honored tradition, but the downside is that it doesn't distinguish muscle from fat—it's just total weight. After all, you can lop your arm off and lose 25 pounds instantly. Instead, combine your body fat measurement with a weight measurement and you'll get a clearer picture of your emerging lean body.

Let me give you an example. Let's say you measure your body fat index using calipers, and it's 25 percent. Next, you hop on a scale, and you weigh 200 pounds.

To figure out how much of your body is fat and how much is lean, do some simple math:

$$\text{Pounds body fat} = \text{body weight} \times \text{body fat index}$$
$$= 200 \times 0.25$$
$$= 50 \text{ pounds fat}$$

Now simply subtract the pounds of body fat from your total weight, and you arrive at how much of you is lean: 150 pounds. Easy, isn't it? By combining these two methods, you can see your results much more clearly than a quick glance in the mirror. See Appendix D for the "Success Tracking Chart."

3. *Unroll the tape measure.* Just take a simple tailor's tape measure and wrap it around your arms, upper thighs, calves, waist, chest, and shoulders to track your progress on a chart from week to week.

4. *Keep track of the weights you're training with.* If you're hoisting 50 pounds one week and then 60 pounds three weeks later—that's some great positive feedback. Relish it. Brag to your friends. You can use the chart on page 198 to note the changes.

5. *Snap photos.* Instead of taking a gander at yourself in the mirror, use photography to measure change. By snapping a few pics at regular intervals during the Lean

Body program, you can gauge your progress. Take front, back, and side photos at the same location and same distance from the camera.

Why photos? Because while sometimes we forget, photographs don't. It's easy to get frustrated and think you're not changing fast enough. But the photographs might reveal quite the opposite—you're making stellar gains, and faster than you think.

Limit your measurements to one time per week to smooth out natural daily physical fluctuations and get a more accurate gauge of your progress.

Get Out Your Pen! (Part III) 🖉

You've written your goals. You've written your self-affirmations. Your third writing assignment, class? Your calendar and training log, which can be found in the Appendixes at the back of this book.

After you've read Part Five ("The Workout"), write down the days you plan to work out over the next 12 weeks (see the Monthly Workout Success Planner on pages 204–05). You'll find that you're more accountable when you keep track of your workouts on a calendar. Plus, there's immense satisfaction in checking workouts off. Each time you tick one off, it is cause for celebration.

You might also want to keep a training journal to track what kinds of exercises you're doing, how you felt on a particular day, what you ate, or any number of subject factors (see the Daily Workout Success Planner on pages 198–99). If you're that detail-oriented, I highly encourage you to put a few minutes aside each day to keep this journal. At the end of each week, you'll be able to review the log and see patterns that might be helpful.

Step #5: Make Failure Work for You

Failing is not a terminal condition. It's a process. How we interpret failures and act upon them ultimately determines whether we persist in, and exist in, failure. Or overcome our temporary obstacles to become a success.

What do I mean by failure is a process? Failure is not a permanent condition unless we let it become a permanent condition.

What does that mean? When achievers fail, they see it only as a momentary blip on the radar, not a lifelong pattern. They don't beat themselves up with self-defeating talk. They refuse to think of themselves as failures. Remember the power of positive self-talk? This is how achievers do it: taking the negatives and either squashing them outright or flipping them around.

Motivation Tip #5

One setback doesn't mean the end of the road. In fact, failure can be the most powerful weapon in your arsenal—if you know how to harness its power. Setbacks are just opportunities in disguise.

Never tell yourself: *I am a failure.* Instead say, *I have failed this one time. But I am going to do something about it.* The question is not whether you will have problems, because you will. It's how you deal with your problems when they arise that will determine your results. At those times you fail, you have to fight negative self-talk. Instead of dwelling on it, say, *I can do better than this. Now I'm going to rebound and get back on track!* If you blow your diet or skip a workout, don't get down, just pick up where you left off.

With a lifestyle change like the Lean Body Promise, the little screwups and steps backward mean less. In the grand scheme of things, it's just not that devastating.

Okay—Put Away Your Pen!

I asked you to do a lot of writing in this chapter. Now you can relax and put the pen away. I have one last thing for you to write, but you won't need ink.

I want you to think about writing your goals into your heart. What do I mean by that? To truly assimilate a goal, you have to do more than write it down on a piece of paper. You have to practice the motivational keys in this book on a daily basis. Together, positive self-affirmation and physical feedback can change your entire outlook on your physical—and mental—life. These tools will help you to internalize and strengthen your desires. And once you strongly desire that goal—when you want it more than you want to return to your old habits—you can consider it written in your heart.

Finally, there's another way to write something into your heart: connect it to people who are already in your heart.

If you have a significant other or a family depending on you, it's vital that you take care of yourself. If you break down, your whole family is at risk. If you don't want to do it for yourself, do it for your family. Do it because looking good and feeling healthy will make you happier in your relationships and more productive at work; you'll inspire others to do the same.

In fact, I encourage you to share this book with a friend or a neighbor. You, too, can be a "fitness evangelist." When you help those around you change their lives for the better, you reap the rewards tenfold in your own life. I know—this is probably the oldest life lesson in the book. But it is completely true. I can't tell you how overjoyed I am to be doing this for a living, and that you're here right now, ready to make this journey with me.

PART FOUR

The Meal Plan

Tuck the napkin into the top of your shirt. Grab your fork and knife. It's time to eat. And believe me—with the Lean Body Meal Plan, you're going to be doing a *lot* of eating.

What? Can that be right? Maybe you've just flipped back to the cover of this book, just to make sure you haven't accidentally picked up an Emeril Lagasse cookbook by mistake. Don't worry. This is still *The Lean Body Promise*, and I'm still talking about how you can lose pounds of fat. But I'm willing to bet you didn't expect that I'd be telling you that in order to lose weight, you're going to have to eat more than you've ever eaten before.

Of course, the plan isn't all about eating. Nutrition and exercise are like the two wheels of a bicycle: if both are in good working order, the bike will take you anywhere you want to go. However, if one or the other is out of commission, you'll be stuck on your front porch. It's the same with your body. Nutrition and exercise work hand in hand to build muscle, burn body fat, and increase health and energy. The Lean Body Promise is based on the principle of Banex (balanced exercise and nutrition). In this section, you'll learn how to eat—more than you think—so that you fuel your fat-burning machine to get the fastest results possible. You'll learn how to balance protein, carbohydrates, and fat to make powerful, body-transforming meals.

The Lean Body Meal Plan is simple enough to be followed for the rest of your life—there's no weighing out or measuring foods. Get ready to enjoy what may possibly be the most user-friendly metabolism-building nutrition program ever. You'll never have to guess what to eat again. And you'll never go hungry again.

Forget Everything You Know About Eating

Let's say you live a sedentary life—office cubicle by day, futon parked in front of the TV by night with potato chips and pilsner of cold beer at your side. As a result, you've become . . . well, to use the polite term, *weight-challenged*. Who should you blame? You could point a finger at fast-food companies and junk food manufacturers for producing the stuff that made you the person (and a half) you are today. You might blame the government for not giving you clear guidance about living a healthy lifestyle. Or you might blame modern society for encouraging lives full of instant gratification and sedentary work and entertainment. You might even turn that finger around at yourself and say, *Gee, maybe I didn't need to finish that whole bag of sour cream and onion potato chips in one sitting.*

If you blame any of the above targets, you'd be wrong. Want to know who to blame? Your own body.

Not *you*. Your *body*. There is a distinction. Your body has a different agenda than you do. Your goals might include being a productive member of society, having fun, looking and feeling great, and occasionally putting yourself in a position to perpetuate the species. Your body? It doesn't give two hoots about any of that, except maybe that last one. No, your body has a single item on its to-do list: Survive. And sometimes, your goals conflict with that singular goal.

In short, your body wants to gather up as much food as possible and eat it all. What it can't use right away will be stored in the form of fat. Your body doesn't know where its next meal is coming from. It has no idea there's a fully stocked supermarket right down the street, or a refrigerator full of food in the kitchen. Your body is not exactly smart. In fact, it's pretty much the biochemical equivalent of Forrest Gump.

In prehistoric times, it was feast or famine, and those who survived were those best adept at storing energy for times of famine. To get you to eat the high-calorie foods necessary for survival, your body releases an opiate-like chemical called dopamine in the brain whenever you eat foods with a high caloric value. It's a drug reward, pure and simple.

The problem is, here in the modern world, we don't need to store food as fat. We can't turn off these survival mechanisms, even though we have an abundant food supply. Your body wants to store fat for winter; you want to look good in that new pair of jeans you bought. Your body wants you to hit that fast-food drive-thru and polish it off at home with a Twinkie; you want to make sure you're able to attract a member of the opposite sex.

What are you supposed to do?

Isn't it true that if I eat less, I'll get thinner?

A number of bad things will happen if you stop eating. Your blood sugar level will plummet, and that triggers your appetite. You'll get cravings. If you don't eat for a long enough time, your survival mechanism kicks in, and your metabolism will slow to conserve energy. You'll turn into a machine with one mission: Find the next meal. People make this mistake all the time when they say, *I don't understand. I'm exercising, I'm not eating, and I'm still fat.* They're missing the point.

Why You Should Start Bouncing Checks

You have to outsmart your body. After all, you're the mind, right? Your body is just an organic mechanism of muscle, bone, tissue, skin, blood, water, and hair. Let's show the body who's boss.

To outsmart your body, it's important to know how it operates. In many ways, your body acts like a bank account. By eating food, you're making a deposit of calories. (A calorie is basically a unit of measurement that represents the energy value of food. Calories are like dollars: without them, your bank account (your body) will cease to function.) Then your metabolism—the number of calories it takes to keep your heart beating, lungs working, all of the cells in your body going, and your brain running—makes periodic withdrawals. And exercising is like writing a big, fat check.

The secret is getting those calorie checks to bounce. Unlike in finance, you actually *want* to be overdrawn, because your body will turn around and pull up calories from your fat stores. And that will make you lose weight. Your body won't have a chance to store up those extra calories, because there won't be any extra calories. It'll have to make do with what you give it, and eventually, it'll have to learn to trust that you're not going to let the two of you starve.

Fitness and nutrition experts call this condition of being overdrawn a "caloric deficit" (hypocaloric). This is a rare situation where a deficit is a good thing. You don't want to alarm your body, because then it will go into survival mode, slowing down your thyroid gland, freezing your metabolism, and messing with your brain until life becomes unpleasant. The goal is just a *slight* deficit, one that will continue until optimal weight is achieved. Nutritionally speaking, you always want to be slightly in the red.

Metabolism is a word that's tossed around a lot, and people have weird ideas about it. If they're overweight, they assume that they were just born with a bad metabolism. Or if they had a kickin' metabolism in college—one that allowed them to snarf cheese fries left and right without gaining an ounce—they assume they lost it sometime in adulthood. Except for rare cases, this simply isn't true. Most people have perfectly fine metabolisms. They just have poor eating habits and don't exercise. These people are letting their body do the meal planning and, as a result, are sabotaging their natural fat-burning systems.

How do you rev up your metabolism so you can become the calorie- and fat-burning machine you were at 17? *The key is building muscle.* Muscle isn't just there to lift boxes when you're helping a friend move, or to impress small children. It's metabolically active tissue, which is a fancy way of saying it burns tons of calories even when it's not doing a darn thing. You want a lot of muscle because that will help you burn fat even when you're just sitting there watching Jay Leno.

THE SKINNY SO FAR . . .

▌ Your body is like a bank account: you make deposits (calories) and withdrawals (bodily functions and exercise).

▌ A caloric deficit—a state in which you burn more calories than you take in—will help you shed extra pounds.

▌ Think you have a bad metabolism? It's probably just fine. Your eating and exercise habits are what need revving up.

▌ Your muscles are your own natural fat-burning machines. Give them the right fuel, give them the exercise they need, and they'll do half the work for you.

Ready to Eat?

The foods and eating patterns in the Lean Body Meal Plan feed lean muscle tissue, which is the metabolic furnace of your body. But the plan also starves your fat stores at the same time. In other words, you'll be able to burn fat while eating more food. In fact, a few days into the Lean Body Meal Plan, you're not going to believe how much food you're expected to eat. *This is a diet?* you might ask yourself. It sounds too good to be true. But it *is* true. When you pair it with your Lean Body Exercise Plan in the next part, you are going to transform yourself into a body fat–burning machine. Your calorie-craving body will never know what hit it.

First, let's see if you're up for the challenge. I have four simple questions to ask you. If you can answer *yes* to all of the following, I hereby pronounce you ready to start the Lean Body Meal Plan. Here goes:

1. *Would you like to eat more often during the day?* This is not a trick question. You'll have to go from eating three squares to eating five smaller meals spread out through the day. (That means three main meals and two mini-meals.) You'll still have breakfast, lunch, and dinner, but you'll add a high-protein snack in the middle of the morning and the afternoon.

    Still with us? How about . . .

2. *Can you eat more protein-packed foods, such as chicken breasts and fish?* And there are many more protein foods to choose from, including ones that are extremely easy to prepare.

    No problem, right? Here's another one:

3. *Can you cut back on sugary desserts?* Okay, maybe this question gives you pause. Visions of sugarplums (and 3 Musketeers bars) might be dancing in your head. But don't worry: you won't be going cold turkey. You'll still be allowed to have your favorite snacks, only less frequently. For example, if you enjoy a Snickers bar four or five times a week, I'm talking about cutting back to one or two per week.

    That's not so bad, right? Just one more question:

4. *Can you cut back on fatty foods and junk food?* Don't panic; you'll be able to replace snacks like potato chips, cookies, and ice cream with healthier versions. (And if the healthy versions don't quite do it for you, you can still have these snacks occasionally.)

If you've said *yes* to all four questions, congrats! You're ready to take the next step. The good news is that the Lean Body Meal Plan is so simple, you'll be able to begin tomorrow. Or even later tonight, if you can make a quick trip to your favorite supermarket to pick up some basics.

By the second week of this program, your body will have already switched over to fat-burning mode. You will not be hungry. Ready to get started?

Choosing Lean Body Foods

All you've got to remember about healthy eating is what, how much, and when. First, let's look at what you'll be eating on the Lean Body Program. Imagine your dinner plate divided into thirds:

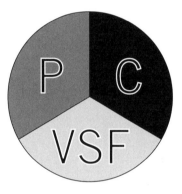

Rule of Thirds
Cover $\frac{1}{3}$ of your plate with a protein,
$\frac{1}{3}$ with a carb, and
the final $\frac{1}{3}$ with a vegetable, salad, or fruit.

P = Protein Foods   C = Carbohydrate Foods   VSF = Vegetables, Salads, and Fruit

The first wedge will hold your protein: the most important part of every meal. No matter what, always make sure there's protein on your plate. The second wedge will hold your carbohydrates. Important note: Not all carbs are evil incarnate, and the right ones can actually help you burn fat. The third wedge will hold vegetables, salad, and fruit. And, yes, there will be a little room for good fats.

The Lean Body Meal Plan is based on the balanced intake of the three major categories of nutrients found in food: protein, carbohydrates, and fats. These nutrients, known as *macronutrients,* supply the material your body needs for energy and repair. The Lean Body Meal Plan is moderate in complex carbohydrates, moderate in protein, and low in fat. Planning a Lean Body meal or mini-meal is as simple as choosing foods from each of these categories and arranging them on your plate in thirds. Let's talk about each of these parts in a bit more depth.

Protein: Muscle Food

Protein builds muscle, so the Lean Body Meal Plan includes plenty of protein. It's important to build your meal plan with a foundation of protein because protein stabilizes blood sugar (thereby easing cravings), feeds muscle tissue, and revs up your metabolism. It is also the only macronutrient that supplies nitrogen, which your muscles need to function properly.

Here's your Lean Body protein list. (The fish with asterisks contain higher levels of fat.)

egg whites or egg substitutes
chicken breast
turkey breast
lean ground turkey breast
bluefish*
cod
crab
flounder
grouper
haddock
halibut
mackerel*
mahi-mahi

orange roughy*

pike

pollack

red snapper

salmon*

scallops

shrimp

sole

swordfish*

tuna*

fat-free cottage cheese

protein powder (CarbWatchers ProPlete, ProV60)

Lean Body Meal Replacement Powder (MRP) Packets, Ready-to-Drink (RTD)
    Shakes, and Bars

Fat-free cottage cheese is great because it contains casein, a milk protein that moves through the body slowly and satiates your appetite. Casein is also very high in amino acids that support muscle tissue and prevent its breakdown. Egg Beaters are another great source of protein. They're egg substitutes that look just like real scrambled eggs.

You'll want to be careful with oily fish, such as salmon, while you're just starting out—there's a bit more fat than other fish. Personally I don't eat oily fish more than a couple times a week. Even though it's loaded with healthy essential fats, you still have to watch the calories.

There are some sources of protein you want to avoid. Beef is way overconsumed in this country. If you need your meat fix, choose the leanest cuts—but keep in mind that only a small handful of cuts fall into that category. You should limit fatty sources of protein, including beef, pork, lamb, and other meat products, because of their high content of unhealthy saturated fats.

Carbs: Brains and Brawn Fuel

Carbohydrates need a better public relations team.

There is no macronutrient that's been more vilified than poor old carbs. Even fat—the nutritional super-villain—has enjoyed a popularity boost in recent years, thanks to fawning cover stories in *The New York Times Magazine* and the *Wall Street Journal.* But all carbs have been heaped into the same evil category and blamed for the weight epidemic that's rolling across the nation.

That's a shame, because your brain runs on carbs. The old gray noodle needs a certain amount of glucose—a fancy term for the sugar found in your blood—to function properly. If it's not getting it from carbs in your diet, your body will start breaking down protein, and the easiest protein to break down is muscle. And as we've discussed, muscle is the metabolic furnace that's going to help you lose the fat. So if you are eliminating carbs, you're basically breaking down your own fat-burning machines.

When you eat carbohydrates, your body produces a hormone called insulin to help keep your blood sugar within a certain range. But insulin also happens to be a powerful fat storage hormone, so your body stores the excess sugar as fat. For fat loss, it is desirable to keep your insulin levels low and stable.

Low-carb diets such as the Atkins Plan seem to "succeed" by accident; it's insulin management by default. Get rid of the carbs—and by extension, much of the sugar—and of course your body won't need to release as much insulin.

The truth is not all carbs are bad. Simple carbs—like cakes, white bread, crackers, cookies, and products made from refined flour and sugar—yeah, they deserve the bad rap. Be my guest. Slap their faces on wanted posters and hunt them down. But complex carbs—yams, lentils, corn, rice—are unfairly tarred with the same brush. These good carbs will not only give you the energy you need all day long, they'll also help you burn fat.

What separates good carbs from the bad? Simple (bad) carbs are converted to sugar very quickly. Those bad boys hit the ground running. That's because simple carbs, if you were to examine them at a molecular level, have a lot of surface area, which make them easy to break down. Complex carbs, on the other hand, don't have as much surface area, so they require more digestion and are broken down more slowly. The release of sugar into the bloodstream is slowed considerably, which means that insulin levels remain lower.

By eating protein with your complex carbs you'll slow the carb-to-fat conversion process even more. This is why you should never eat complex carbs alone; always pair them with protein.

Here's your Lean Body complex carb list. You should limit the carbs denoted with an asterisk:

oatmeal
whole-grain cooked cereal
Cream of Wheat
brown rice
wild rice
new potatoes (with skin)
sweet potatoes
yams
beans
corn

peas
rice cakes
lentils
black-eyed peas
whole-grain pasta and bread*
corn tortillas

There is still another way of slowing down the release of carb sugar into your bloodstream. It's a method that has been handed down through the generations, and was most often uttered by your mother at the kitchen table: "Eat your vegetables."

How Carbs Became the Enemy

Blame it on the 1980s.

If you were around back then, you'll remember that the low-fat diet was all the craze. Fat was the enemy and needed to be eliminated with extreme prejudice. So what was left? Protein and carbs. Food manufacturers went crazy with the latter, introducing all kinds of low-fat products. The low-fat cookie. The low-fat snack cake. The low-fat pastry strudel. The low-fat plate of funnel cake.

Let's take that pastry strudel, for example. The package claims that it's 95 percent fat-free. Sounds good, right? The strudel may not be high in fat, but it's loaded with sugar from simple carbs, which means more fat storage. In the '80s and '90s, people became fat by overrelying on carbs. Hence, carbs got a bad name.

Essential Fats: The Friendly Fats

The last component of our Lean Body Meal Plan is fat. Put down the holy water and crucifix. Fat is not quite the monster the ultralow-fat bunch think it is.

Fat intake might sound like a strange part of a diet plan, but I like to tell people they need to become fat conscious (aware of the fat content of their foods). As with carbs, there are good and bad fats. Bad fats contain large amounts of partially saturated, saturated, and trans-fatty acids. You find these in processed and fried foods, beef, pork, lamb, cheese, cream, and butter. Want a shock? Pick up the packages of your favorite foods and scan the nutrition panels. Anything that is more than 20 percent fat by calories means you'll be overloading your body with more fat than you want. (I'll explain more about reading these panels for fat content a little further along.)

Good fats, on the other hand, usually contain essential fatty acids (EFAs), which our bodies can't make on their own, and which play a role in virtually every function in the body.

Here are examples of healthy fats:

flaxseed oil
salmon, mackerel, sardines
fish oils
walnuts, almonds, cashews, other nuts and seeds
avocadoes
olive oil
olives

You can still get chubby on good fats. They're not free foods by any stretch. But in small amounts, they're an important part of your diet. Unfortunately, many good fats naturally found in our food supply are destroyed during processing and cooking. To make sure you're getting enough good fats in your diet, add a tablespoon of flaxseed oil, olive oil, or a small handful of nuts to two or three of your daily meals. A slice of avocado works great also.

It's really important to avoid the bad fats—especially animal fats, as well as any other processed foods that are high in trans-fatty acids—while on the Lean Body Meal Plan. These foods can wreak havoc on your health. Here are some examples of what to **avoid**:

luncheon meats
red meat
pork
cheese
butter
margarine
egg yolks
sour cream
salad dressings
fries
chips
ice cream
mayonnaise
chocolate

The good news: there are plenty of substitutes for them. (See page 84 for ideas.)

>> How much fat is in this thing, anyway?

With the Lean Body Meal Plan, your fat calorie intake is limited to less than 20 percent of total calories for the day. This means you have to be careful to watch out for hidden fats if you eat packaged food. Here's an easy formula to figure out the percentage of fat in any given food. First, look on the "Nutrition Facts" panel of the package, then do a little math:

1. Take the grams of "fat per serving" and multiply by 9. If there are 10 grams of fat, you've got 90 fat calories. (Fat contains 9 calories per gram.)

2. Divide those fat calories by the "total number of calories per serving." Let's say there are 200 calories in a serving. Divide 90 by 200, and you get 45 percent. This means that the product in your hands is essentially 45 percent fat calories. Yikes. Put down the strudel.

But you don't need a calculator. It's possible to guesstimate right there in the supermarket. As long as you have your two vital numbers (total calories and the calories from fat), you can quickly figure out the fat content. If the total calories are 100, it's easy; the fat calories number will be your percentage. For example:

50 calories

5 calories from fat

That's not so bad. Double the 50 to get 100, then double the 5 to get 10, and you realize that this food is only 10 percent fat calories. In general, the greater the distance between the two numbers, the better. But for example:

300 calories

260 calories from fat

There's no doubt about it here—you've got a high-fat food, and you didn't even have to add a single digit. That's because the two numbers are very close. With some practice, reading labels will become second nature. Plus, it also helps pass the time during those trips to the supermarket.

Salad and Vegetables: Free Food

It's no wonder Mom was always pushing the veggies. Vegetables are fibrous carbohydrates with very little in the way of useable calories, so they don't count when adding up a day's worth of calories. In other words, you can eat all you want. They're filling, so your appetite will be satiated longer. They slow down the digestive process, which means that the absorption of carbohydrates becomes even more gradual, which is good for the fat-burning process. In doing that, fiber helps keep your blood sugar stable and your insulin under control.

You eat fiber, but your body doesn't absorb it. (In some ways, you're only renting that bowl of fiber flakes you ate for breakfast.) Fiber's main job is to take a trip through your body, grabbing as much junk and fatty acids and other nasty deposits as it can, then pass safely through the other side. Think of fiber as "nature's Brillo pad," scrubbing your intestines clean as it works its way through your body. Clean intestines means you'll be able to absorb more of the nutrients and vitamins from the healthy food you're eating.

Here's your vegetable list. I call them "free foods," because you can eat as much as you want:

lettuce and leafy greens
broccoli
cauliflower
green beans
carrots
spinach
asparagus
artichokes
peppers
tomatoes
peas
cabbage

zucchini

cucumbers

squash

onions

mushrooms

Frozen vegetables are better than canned, because the canned variety tend to be soggy and salted, whereas their frozen brethren are simply picked, flash-frozen, and then sent to the supermarket. But fresh veggies are best—and steaming is the best way to cook them.

Fruits: Lean Body Desserts

The easiest, most transportable, and tastiest dessert you can eat is fruit. These aren't free foods like vegetables; there's still a lot of natural sugars in these little guys. But they're also high in fiber, which slows down their absorption. If you keep it down to two to three servings per day—maybe a midmorning snack and an after-dinner dessert—you'll manage to satisfy your sugar cravings without resorting to fatty, sugar-laden, overprocessed junk. Hit the supermarket or local farmers' market and stock up on a week's worth of

cherries

grapefruit

berries (blue, black, rasp, straw)

peaches

apricots

oranges

pears

plums

tangerines

apples
grapes*
raisins*
mangoes*
melons (cantaloupe, honeydew)*
dates*
figs*
pineapples*
bananas*

Fruits marked with an asterisk are higher in sugar, and hence should be eaten sparingly. If you're worried that your potato chip fix can't be satisfied with a handful of blueberries, relax. There are alternative snack options, and you'll find them in our trip to the snack aisle of the supermarket on page 92.

Won't I miss all of that sugar and fat?

I have two bits of good news for you: for one, you shouldn't feel deprived, because in the Lean Body plan, you'll be allowed to "cheat" twice a week. You're not saying good-bye to sugar and fat altogether. You're just controlling how much you eat.

The other good news is that your taste buds are willing to be retrained. It only takes two or three weeks before they forget about all of the sugar-laden stuff you used to eat and start to enjoy the healthy food you're now treating yourself to. The interesting thing is that the longer you make the Lean Body Promise part of your daily routine, the less you'll crave sugar and fat.

Just Add Water

There's one last thing to add to your meal plan: water. Like sea monkeys, human beings need water to thrive. You should drink at least two cups of water with every meal. That adds up to a minimum of 10 cups of pure, fresh water each day. You should also get into the habit of sipping water while you work, play, or exercise. Why? Since you'll be doing so much fat-burning, toxins might be released from your stores of body fat. Water helps flush these toxins out of our body. Water increases your satiety level, making you feel less hungry. Water is also essential in every metabolic function in the human body—after all, muscles are 75 percent water.

You'll also want to choose water instead of sugary soft drinks, which can erase your hard-earned gains one 12-ounce can at a time. (For more, see page 93, "Carbonation and Booze City.")

Vitamins, Minerals, and Protein Supplements

Vitamins, minerals, and protein supplements will be very helpful to you on the Lean Body program. As the name implies, supplements . . . er, *supplement* your diet and make it easier to get all of the nutrients your body needs. But they are not substitutes for balanced nutrition.

Vitamins and minerals are nutrients that you require to regulate the functioning of your cells, the conversion of food into energy, and the strengthening and maintenance of everyday physiological processes. They can be found in natural, unprocessed foods such as fruits and vegetables.

But the vitamin content of fruits and vegetables is sometimes compromised by modern mass production methods. Crops are often grown in soil that has been depleted of minerals through overuse. If that's not bad enough, most foods are overprocessed or overcooked, leaving them stripped of their natural nutrients. Just to be on the safe side, you should take a good multivitamin-multimineral supplement derived from natural sources with breakfast every morning. This will help you to feel more energy and help you recover better from exercise.

Protein supplements are beneficial because they make it easy to get high-quality protein at meals without a lot of preparation. They can help you to stay in compliance with your nutrition program. Protein supplements generally fall into four categories: protein powders, meal replacement powders (MRP), ready-to-drink protein shakes (RTD), and protein bars.

Protein powders are usually mixed in a blender with skim milk, water, or fruit juice to make a protein drink. MRPs come in handy, premeasured packets, and often also contain carbs, fats, vitamins, and minerals, to make for a more complete mini-meal. RTD shakes are premixed and come in individual serving size containers that you just open and drink. Choose shakes in soft-side drink boxes, as the canned variety are often overcooked during processing. Protein bars are delicious alternatives to candy bars and desserts, but don't overdo them. Some are high in sugar and fat.

My personal favorites are RTD shakes, because of their nutrition and convenience. Shakes are handy when you need concentrated nutrition and you don't have time to prepare a meal. (See Appendix A on page 195.)

Be wary of over-the-counter diet and fat-burning pills and other supplements that promise benefits that seem too good to be true. They often are, and will serve to lighten only your wallet or purse. Balanced exercise and nutrition (Banex) is the key to your Lean Body success.

I Protein is the building block of every Lean Body meal because it stabilizes your blood sugar, slows down the absorption of other foods, and helps build your muscles.

I Not all carbs are evil, no matter what the trendiest low-carb diets say. Your brain and muscles need them in moderation to function. But there are such things as good and bad carbs; the Lean Body Meal Plan helps you steer clear of the bad and enjoy just the right amount of the good.

I Fat's not necessarily evil, either—if you know how to choose good fats, such as those found in fish and nuts.

I On the Lean Body Meal Plan, you can eat all of the salads and vegetables you want and snack on low-calorie fruit.

How Much to Eat?

You have the **what**. Now it's time for the "how much" part of our meal plan. First, I'll give you the scientific method, just in case you prefer numbers. For the rest of us, there is a no-brainer way to make sure you're dishing out the correct proportions.

1. Protein

You need about 1 gram of protein per pound of body weight. Let's say you're a 200-pound guy. The math is easy: 1 gram × 200 pounds = 200 grams of protein per day, divided in equal amounts over five meals. That works out to about 40 grams of protein per meal. If you're a 140-pound woman, it would be 140 grams. (Thankfully, this isn't rocket science.) Protein contains 4 calories in every gram. So if you require 200 grams of protein, you need 800 calories from protein every day.

> *Or you can skip all the math and keep in mind my favorite rule:*
> *The portion of protein at primary meals (breakfast, lunch, dinner)*
> *should be the size of the palm of your open hand.*

Go ahead. Hold this book with one hand, then look at your other hand. Imagine your fingers and thumb disappearing. Now imagine your palm magically transforming into a delicious piece of orange roughy. There's your protein. (Note: Please be careful to transform your imaginary orange roughy back into your palm before reading any further; you don't want fish stains on the pages.)

2. Carbohydrates

You need about 1 to 1.5 grams of complex carbs per pound of body weight. Crunch the numbers, and you'll see that our 200-pound guy needs 200 to 300 grams of carbs per day, and our woman needs about 140 to 200 grams. Carbs also contain 4 calories per gram, so if you do the math, our guy needs about 800 to 1,200 carb calories per day, and our woman needs about 560 to 800 carb calories.

> *But you can forget that if you remember that your serving of*
> *complex carbs at primary meals (breakfast, lunch, dinner)*
> *should be about the size of your fist.*

I don't have to make you magically transform your fist into a sweet potato, do I? You get the picture. And with palms and fists, you're already two-thirds of the way there.

What If I'm "Carb-Phobic"?

If you feel that you are really sensitive to carbohydrates, I suggest the following: simply eat your "fists of carbs" at the three main meals of the day (breakfast, lunch, and dinner) and stick with a protein bar or shake—and no carbs—during your midmorning and mid-afternoon mini-meals.

3. Vegetables and Salad

Good news: no measuring required! You can have as much of these foods as you like. But remember the rule of thirds, and aim to have this portion be about a third of your total plate.

4. Fat

Add one tablespoon of flaxseed oil or olive oil to your salad or vegetables, and you've got it covered. Or maybe you prefer to get your fat from avocadoes, nuts, seeds, or fish—salmon, for instance, doubles as protein and essential fat.

5. Fruit

Have a small serving of low-calorie fruit at two or three of your meals for dessert. Or, you may prefer a scoop of sorbet at lunch or dinner.

Mix and match from the lists of Lean Body foods, and you have the makings of perfect fat-burning meals.

>> On Preparing Food

You'll notice that none of the recipes in this book (starting on page 215) use the words *oil*, *fry*, *butter*, or *gobs of bacon fat*. That's because none of the Lean Body food you enjoy should be prepared this way. Always bake, steam, broil, or grill your food, and opt for healthy seasonings—herbs, spices, lemons, balsamic vinegar— that will amplify the taste without amplifying your waist.

When to Eat

As with Hollywood careers and paintball skirmishes, timing is everything. The number of times you eat in a day can mean the difference between succeeding or failing on the Lean Body program. **You need to eat five small meals per day**—in other words, a meal every three hours. Why so frequently? By eating small, frequent meals, you never get hungry enough to pig out. Think of it as eating three primary meals (breakfast, lunch, and dinner) with a midmorning snack and midafternoon mini-meal in between.

Your primary meals should be sit-down affairs whenever possible. These three meals should incorporate a plate of food divided into thirds. The midmorning and midafternoon mini-meals can be protein-based snacks such as a protein shake, a protein bar, or a cup of fat-free cottage cheese along with a piece of fruit and small handful of nuts.

Your body can only utilize so many nutrients at one time, so many calories in one sitting. To prevent your body from depositing extra calories as body fat, we've got to parcel out the calories in small, equal amounts during the day. Eating every three hours will also bathe your muscles in nutrients and amino acids.

Unfortunately, the American idea of "three squares a day" is a recipe for disaster— even if you're making a conscious attempt to eat healthy.

Maybe you start the day with just a cup of hot coffee. *Cool*, you figure, *I'm saving calories right there.* And maybe lunch is nothing but a salad with dressing. *That's healthy, right?* Then comes dinner, which is a marathon session of 2,000 or even 3,000 calories in one sitting. *But I deserve it, right? I haven't eaten all day.* Bad move. Remember: Your body is only capable of using so many calories at a time. If you pounded down 3,000 calories of food at one sitting, and your body was only able to use 500 of those calories, guess where the other 2,500 calories are going? Places that don't look so great when you wear a bathing suit. By eating in this manner, you effectively starve your body all day (famine) followed by overeating (feast). You're training your body to deposit fat.

On the other hand, eating five 600-calorie meals changes the game completely. You're only giving your body as much as it can use at one time, leaving no leftovers to store. Think of it as establishing trust with your body. *See? There's more food coming. In fact, food shows up every three hours. Isn't that great? There's no need to store anything! Now put down that clump of fat cells, nice and easy.*

How will I feel during the first week of the Lean Body Meal Plan?

After you get through the first couple of weeks of this program, you'll feel energy all the time. That's because, as we've seen earlier, your body is running optimally. The downside is that you might experience a bit of crankiness at first. Remember: Your brain wants to reward you for eating food with the highest caloric value. That means junk. So, for a few days, you might be irritable. But it won't take long for you to adjust.

Keep Fat Out of the Storage Bin (i.e., Your Spare Tire)

There's another good reason for eating these low-fat, protein-carb-vegetable meals five times a day: you'll be taking advantage of your body's *thermic effect*. When you eat, you're not just adding calories, you're actually burning calories, too, as your body works hard to digest what you've eaten.

This is why the Lean Body program makes such a big deal about these macronutrients. Some foods have a greater thermic effect than others. It's hard to get fat on protein, because protein requires more calories to digest than both of the other two macronutrients put together. And if your body wants to store excess protein calories, it has to go through a three-step process. First, protein has to be broken down into amino acids. Second, amino acids have to be converted to sugars. And lastly, excess sugars are deposited as fat.

Carbohydrates, on the other hand, are easier to digest. They're only two steps away from becoming fat deposits. And fat is . . . well, fat. One tiny step, and you'll be wearing that donut; if you don't use the fat you eat right away, it's going right into that storage bin. That's why you should keep fat calories low. Salad and vegetables are considered free because they require more calories to digest than they contain.

How to Cheat

Too many diets are "all-or-nothing" diets. A strict, Spartan plan, no matter how well intentioned, is destined for failure. On the Lean Body plan, I encourage you to stay within the guidelines, but twice a week you can "cheat" at a meal and enjoy a small portion of your favorite foods. It's what I call a "cheat meal." Follow the Lean Body Meal Plan all day Monday and Tuesday, then by Wednesday night, you're allowed a cheat meal. And then again on Saturday. It works out to about every fourth day. Many people tend to crave these kinds of foods at dinner, but you can cheat at either lunch or dinner.

When you cheat, always start your meal with a protein serving, no matter what.

The protein will stabilize your blood sugar and feed your muscles with amino acids. That way, whatever comes next—a taco, a handful of fries, a wedge of cheesecake—the damage is minimized. Once you've eaten that protein and fed your muscles, your appetite will already be partly satisfied. Never cheat when you're hungry, because you'll tend to overeat. Don't overdo cheating, because it can wipe out a week's worth of dieting.

➤➤ Craving This? Eat *This* Instead

There are often healthy substitutes for your old standbys. The best substitutes are always fresh fruit or raw vegetables. But when you absolutely have a craving, you can find a healthier choice. Here are some of my favorites:

CRAVING *THIS?*	EAT *THIS...*
Chocolate ice cream	Low-fat ice cream, sorbet, frozen yogurt
Neapolitan sundae	Frozen yogurt topped with mixed fruit sorbet
Cheese curls	Hard or thin pretzels
Chips and dip	Low-fat tortilla chips and salsa
Cheese and crackers	Fat-free cottage cheese and rice cakes
Candy bar	Lean Body Gold or CarbWatcher's Protein Bar
Donut	Whole-grain bagel with sugar-free strawberry preserves
Potato chips	Baked potato chips or air-popped popcorn
Corn muffin	Whole-grain English muffin
Strawberry shortcake	Fresh strawberries with nonfat whipped topping
Raspberry tart	Fresh raspberries with nonfat whipped topping
Cheeseburger	Soy or veggie burger with lettuce, tomatoes, onions, pickles
Salted peanuts	Raw almonds

Planning Is the Key to Success

I don't blame you for being a little skeptical about your ability to squeeze in five meals a day. After all, the American Way of Eating till Full ("AWE-full") seems to be one big fat meal at the end of the day to take care of the others you missed. We all have increasingly hectic schedules, with responsibilities imposed on us by work, family, and the IRS. And not necessarily in that order.

On Sundays, try to prepare for the entire week ahead. Cook up a big batch of grilled chicken breasts, baked potatoes and yams, rice, beans, and steamed vegetables. Then put individually sized portions (fists, palms; see page 79) into plastic bags and throw them in the fridge or freezer. The potatoes and rice go into the fridge—they don't freeze well. For the chicken, beans, and vegetables, throw half in the fridge (for the first three days) and the rest into the freezer (for the following two days).

Then, every weekday morning, simply reach into the fridge, grab as many bags of grilled chicken, carbs, and veggies as you'll need for the day, and toss them into a cooler. You can also pack a lot of easily transportable snacks: canned tuna, bananas, baked potatoes, yams, packets of oatmeal, and protein shakes.

When you arrive at work, keep the cooler by your desk and pull out food as needed. With a little bit of effort on a Sunday, you'll be set for the week. It's easy. And the meals only take about five minutes to prepare, and 10 to 15 minutes to eat. That means you'll have plenty of time left over to devote to work. There's no wasted time in a drive-thru lane, or trying to demolish a huge submarine sandwich at your desk only to find a brown piece of lettuce in your desk drawer three months later. In fact, the busier you are, the more the Lean Body Meal Plan makes sense.

›› Labrada Family Time-Saver Tips

by Robin Labrada

1. Planning ahead and cooking in quantities can save you time. For example, if you are making rice for dinner, simply make a big pot and store the rest. Making chicken? Make eight breasts instead of two. Baking potatoes? Bake six potatoes and six yams. Use what you need for dinner and throw the rest in the fridge. It's easy.

2. Twice a week, cook more than usual. On Sunday I'll cook for the first part of the week. On Thursday I'll do this again, just with different items. I'll make a pot of brown rice with pecans and cranberries, three yams, five baked potatoes, a pot of soup, six grilled chicken breasts, and a batch of muffins. After everything cools, pop them into individual plastic bags and containers. This usually takes about two hours. Sure, that's a lot of food—but it saves time in the long run. My husband takes three or four meals every day, and all he has to do is grab those little containers and bags and throw them into a cooler.

3. Buy two ready-made roasted chickens instead of one. We'll have one for dinner, and while the other is still warm I'll pull the chicken off the bone, separate it into white and dark meat, put it in bags, and refrigerate them. That way, I'll have fresh chicken—not processed deli meats—for the kids' sandwiches, instant chicken burritos, or grilled cheese and chicken.

4. Skip the heads—buy lettuce in bags. You just grab a bunch, rinse and toss into bowls, and add your favorite dressing and toppings.

A Typical Day on the Lean Body Meal Plan

All the theory in the world is great, but unless you apply it to everyday life, it's completely useless. (Stephen J. Hawking is a smart guy and everything, but when's the last time you used his theories of space and time while driving home from work? Yeah. That's what I thought.) Fortunately, the Lean Body Meal Plan is all about practical applications. Let's walk you through a typical day so you can see how to use the Lean Body Meal Plan every step of the way.

In the morning, start with breakfast. If you're going to skip a meal, this is not the one to skip. When you wake up, your heart rate goes up, your metabolism kicks into high gear, and you get hungry. Studies show that people who take the time to eat a quick breakfast have a higher energy level throughout the day and avoid that midafternoon energy crash.

Next, head to the kitchen, measure out a cup of oatmeal, pour a cup of skim milk on it, then let it sit for 15 minutes. Take your shower or read the paper. By the time you're finished, the oats will be soft. Sprinkle a sugar substitute (I'm fond of Splenda) on top to sweeten it. Or add some cinnamon. That takes care of your carbs. For protein, add a Lean Body Meal Replacement Protein Powder (See Appendix A for more information) to the oatmeal, or mix it into 16 ounces of ice water, which gives you about 40 grams of high-quality protein. Finish it off with a tablespoon of flaxseed oil. It's a simple breakfast that you can eat in less than five minutes.

On weekends, when you have more time, scramble 10 egg whites (or Egg Beaters), add crumbled nonfat tortilla chips, and finish off with salsa on top. This makes a delicious nonfat, high-protein omelet. You might also have a whole-grain muffin for carbs.

Come midmorning, pause in your work and have a cup of fat-free cottage cheese and a granola bar or banana. That will tide you over until lunch, when you can nuke a broiled chicken breast, a baked yam, and one cup of frozen vegetables. If you feel like it, have a piece of fruit, a granola bar, or a handful of nuts for dessert. Midafternoon, enjoy a Lean Body Ready-to-Drink Shake and an apple. Finally, for dinner, sit down and enjoy broiled fish, rice and beans, and vegetables, along with a salad dressed with balsamic vinegar and a tablespoon of olive oil. If you get hungry later in the evening, try fruit, fat-free cottage cheese, protein bars, air-popped popcorn, or rice cakes.

In Appendix E, you will find a detailed 7-day sample meal plan that you can use to structure your daily meals. All of the recipes used in the meal plans can be found in Appendix F. You'll also find a handy Nutrition Success Planner on page 200, which will help you keep track of your day-to-day eating.

THE SKINNY SO FAR . . .

- The fat-loss equation hinges on the macronutrient makeup of the meal plan, the caloric deficit, and meal frequency.

- Lean people tend to be "grazers" who feast on multiple small meals during the day. Not-so-lean people tend to be "stuffers" who starve all day, then gorge on one large meal at day's end.

- An important part of the Lean Body Meal Plan is frequency: for maximum results, you have to eat at least five times a day. This trains your body to use calories as it receives them—and not store them away as fat. Think of your day as the primary meals—breakfast, lunch, and dinner—with two snacks or mini-meals in between. You may also have a snack after dinner, if you get hungry.

- Forget counting calories and instead focus on portions. To estimate how much protein you should eat, look at the palm of your open hand, and serve yourself a similar-sized portion. How much carbs? Make a fist, and do the same.

- Cheating is actually an important part of this plan: if you can avoid the feeling of being deprived, you'll stick with this plan indefinitely. Have two cheat meals per week.

- Prepare meals ahead of time.

LET'S GO SHOPPING

If your refrigerator and cupboard aren't full of Lean Body–friendly foods, you increase your chances of throwing in the towel and calling out for pizza. Remember that planning is a key to success. If you wait until you're hungry to think about what you'll eat, you're setting yourself up for failure.

Let's go on a virtual shopping trip through your average American supermarket. Along the way, we'll try to minimize picking food that comes in boxes and cans and plastic wrap—processed foods. And as you'll see, a little label-reading can make all of the difference.

TERROR IN THE AISLES

Before we head into the automatic sliding front doors, let's discuss two slippery tricks that some food marketers use to make you think you're eating healthy when you're actually not.

1. The Fat Percent Swindle. The front of the package cries out, *Now 95% Fat-Free!* Naturally, you assume that the product is only 5 percent fat; the rest is lean. Hence, it falls within the guidelines of the Lean Body Meal Plan, right?

Wrong.

How is this possible? Let me give an extreme example. Take a cup containing three ounces of water, which has no calories. Next, take a one-ounce piece of butter, which is 100 percent fat calories. Now add one ounce of butter to the water in the cup. Three ounces of water, one ounce of butter. One hundred percent of the calories still come from fat.

But you could sell that and claim it's 75 percent fat free. How? Because that claim is based on weight. Which would be technically true—those three ounces of water don't have a calorie anywhere. But the ounce of butter sure does, and that's 100 percent from fat. This is a trick food manufacturers play all the time.

2. The "Fat-Free" Scam. Here's another diabolical one. One gram of fat has 9 calories. By law, if something has less than a half gram of fat per serving, you can label the product "fat-free." Let's say it's a salad dressing with only 4 calories from fat per tablespoon. The manufacturer labels the product fat-free. What they don't want you to notice is that puny serving size: a single tablespoon. Suddenly, those grams of fat add up. By making the serving size small enough, it's possible to have food labeled fat-free, even if it's 100 percent fat from calories.

AISLE 1A: BAD CARB LAND

The first thing I see is a package of **bagels.** Let's scan the label: 250 calories, with 10 calories from fat, so it qualifies as a low-fat food. There are 5 grams of sugar. Not bad. Still, bagels are not an everyday choice for someone who's trying to lose a lot of fat quickly. If you read the ingredients, you'll see that most are made of enriched bleached flour, which metabolizes very quickly. If you had this bagel with a chicken breast and a salad, and on that salad you had a tablespoon of olive oil or flaxseed oil, it would slow down the absorption of this bagel considerably.

You should limit **bread** consumption. But if you're going to have some, your best bet is bread made from 100 percent whole grains, which means they've used the entire grain. Most other kinds of bread—especially white bread—are made from bleached flour that has had all of the bran removed, and has been bleached white and stripped of all its vitamins and minerals.

AISLE 3B: A COLD CASE

You'll want to stay away from **cold cuts**. The meats are often injected with water and chemicals to retard spoilage, and the fat content tends to be astronomical. And there's enough sodium in these cuts to stun a family of garden slugs. Even healthy-sounding cuts like **oven-prepared turkey breast** can be misleading. A label might say "98% fat-free," but when you look at the label you see that there are 45 total calories, and 10 of them come from fat. Do the math. It's actually 22 percent fat by calories, but says 98 percent fat-free.

Instead, try the **rotisserie-cooked chicken**. It's hot and ready to eat—just skip the skin.

AISLE 4A: THE PROMISED LAND

Everywhere you look, there are plenty of juicy and sweet **fruits** for you to enjoy guilt-free. The only fruits you should watch are those that are higher in sugar, such as tropical fruits: pineapples, bananas, mangoes, and such. But even those are better than reaching for a candy bar or a slice of cake. Fruits have lots of fiber, vitamins, and enzymes.

Likewise, there are dozens of **vegetables** waiting to be picked and bagged. Avocadoes are high in fats, but at least they're healthy fats; eaten in small amounts along with your protein and carbs, they fall within the Lean Body–friendly fat guidelines. Leafy salads are always good, whether you use iceberg lettuce or baby spinach greens. **Potatoes** aren't "free," but if you leave the skin on you'll have the fiber and vitamins you need to digest the starchy inside.

Where people get into trouble is with **salad dressings**. Pick up regular blue cheese dressing and it'll likely have 90 to 100 percent of its calories from fat. Even seemingly healthy picks such as "light ranch dressing" can pack 72 of its 80 calories from fat. Your safest bet is using **balsamic vinegar**. Choose a healthy oil, such as olive or flaxseed, to mix with your balsamic vinegar.

BACK AISLE: DAIRY LAND

Egg whites, as you already know, are fine; you just have to get rid of the yolks. Egg Beaters are recommended, but feel free to use any other kind of egg substitutes, or just crack and strain your own. **Butter** and **margarine** are both 100 percent saturated fat, hence nobody's friend.

Most **liquid "fat-free" coffee creamers** claim to have zero calories from fat, but the ingredients are water, sugar, corn syrup (i.e., more sugar) and partially hydrogenated soybean oil. Wait a second—how is that possible? Since fewer than 9 calories per serving come from fat, they can get away with putting "zero" there. Use low-fat milk or nonfat dry milk for your coffee creamer instead. Since less than a half gram is in a serving, you can get away with "zero."

AISLE 5B: HYDROGENATED HELL

You might have heard the furor over **trans-fat** in the news lately. You have a right to be concerned. This kind of fat is the worst artery-clogging, cancer-causing substance you can put into your body.

You'll know you're dealing with trans-fat if you see the words **hydrogenated** or **partially hydrogenated oil** in the ingredient list of a packaged food. That means food processors took vegetable oil and bubbled hydrogen through it. The result is a solid fat mass. On the upside, the product will stay shelf-worthy for months. On the downside, it raises your cholesterol like an Apollo rocket. And studies have linked trans-fat to cancer.

Cookies are the worst culprits when it comes to hydrogenated oils. Take your chocolate sandwich cookie with a creme filling. The outside is flour and sugar; the inside is pure hydrogenated fat. Both break down easily and convert to stored fat. **Crackers** are nothing more than white flour and hydrogenated oil, packing a hideous amount of fat calories.

Nuts aren't bad, but opt for raw. Anytime fats and oils are heated up, they start breaking down, which is how an otherwise healthy fat can turn into a bad fat. **Popcorn** can be a good snack, too, if you choose the air-popped variety. And **fat-free tortilla chips and salsa** are okay, provided you read the labels to make sure there are no hidden oils somewhere in the salsa.

AISLE 7A: CARBONATION AND BOOZE CITY

Soft drinks are another staple of American culture. Where else in the world could you find a multimillion-dollar corporate war devoted to determining the nation's best soda pop? If you can't stand to live without a can of **soda** now and again, definitely opt for the diet varieties. The fully leaded sodas are usually 100 percent sugar water. (And one can of soda may contain the equivalent of 12 teaspoons of sugar.)

As for more potent drinks: Alcoholic beverages such as **beer**, **wine**, and **cocktails** may be fat-free, but a single gram of alcohol contains about seven calories. Drink one 12-ounce brew, and you're ingesting 150 calories. Plus, alcohol increases your appetite, hardens and clogs your arteries, and slows down your fat-burning process. To see optimal results from your first 12 weeks of the program, keep your alcohol intake to an absolute minimum.

But if you still crave the occasional pint of ale or dry martini, try to select drinks with the lowest alcohol content (proof). The lower the proof, the fewer the calories. An ounce and a half of 80 proof liquor contains 97 calories; the same amount of 100 proof liquor contains 125 calories.

AISLE 9B: DRY GOODS

You don't want to overdo **pasta**. In fact, when you're starting out with the Lean Body Meal Plan, I'd advise you skip it altogether—after all, pasta is simply flour, easily digested and turned into fat stores. Later on, feel free to reintroduce a little of it, but please don't pour Alfredo sauce over it. Go with marinara sauce, and use whole-wheat or soy pasta only, which breaks down more slowly.

Brown (whole-grain) rice contains the bran husk, so it breaks down slower than its bleached counterpart, white rice. The wild rice mixes are pretty complex—and hence, good for your digestive system. **Beans** are awesome. Black beans, red beans, lentils, kidney beans, split peas . . . they're all wonderful, because they pack a lot of protein and fiber. Mix them with rice, and you have one of the best complex carbohydrates going.

AISLE 10A: THE MEAT MARKET

Like carbs, meat shouldn't be demonized. There are good meats, and there are bad. To put it simply, lean meats such as **fish, chicken,** and **turkey** are good; other forms of animal flesh—fatty cuts of beef, pork, or lamb—are not so good.

Depending on the time of year, **tuna** varies in its fat content. Pick up a can of Brand X solid white albacore. Then pick up Brand Z solid white albacore. At first glance, both appear to be the same product. Now take a look at the fat by calories. Brand X turns out to be 45 percent fat. But somehow Brand Z is only 15 percent fat. How? Turns out, these two brands of tuna were caught at different times during the year. If you catch them during the winter, when they're fat, you'll have more calories from fat.

Not all fowl is created equal, either. **Canned white chicken meat** will do in a pinch, but the sodium content is usually sky-high, so be careful. And while **turkey sausage** often claims "lean" on the packaging, those links are usually more than half fat calories. Stick with **white breast meat** when it comes to **chicken** and **turkey**.

If you're going to eat red meat, choose lean cuts of beef and limit it to once per week. Look for the key words: **round** and **loin**. There are seven cuts that are "lean" according to the U.S. Nutrition Labeling and Education Act:

> *eye round* **(4.2 grams of fat)**
> *top round* **(also 4.2 grams)**
> *round tip* **(5.9 grams)**
> *top sirloin* **(6.1 grams)**
> *bottom round* **(6.3 grams)**

top loin (**8.0 grams**)

tenderloin (**8.5 grams**)

All of these cuts, oddly enough, pack less fat than a chicken thigh (which has 9.2 grams of fat). Still, these cuts pale in comparison to a good old **chicken breast**, which has only 3.0 grams of fat.

AISLE 12B: AMBER WAVES OF GRAINS

The best Lean Body–friendly cereal, hands down, is **oatmeal**. Go for whole oats, since they break down more slowly than one-minute oats. (But in a pinch, those will work, too.) Be careful with instant oatmeal, especially the flavored varieties, which can have high sugar and fat content. **Multigrain hot cereal**, **Cream of Wheat**, **barley**, **oat bran**, and **grits** are all smart choices.

Of course, you want to avoid those sugary Saturday-morning kids' cereals that feature cartoon animals or monsters. They shouldn't even be served to children. But even healthy-sounding cereals can be full of hidden fats and sugars. Most packaged **granola** is guilty of packing in serious sugar and fat, especially from the oils used for processing. **Granola bars** are certainly better than candy bars, since the primary ingredient is oats. But that's where it stops, because the next two ingredients tend to be sugar and oil.

How to Order in Restaurants

I t's always preferable to fix your own meals at home because you have control. But sometimes you're faced with situations that require you to eat in public. Like a business lunch. (Or your wedding day.) When you absolutely, positively have to have someone else do the cooking—or just want to enjoy a night out without breaking your Lean Body Promise—keep these handy rules in mind.

1.	*If it's a business lunch, offer to make the reservation.* That way, you can choose a restaurant you know offers Lean Body–friendly food. If someone else is doing the choosing, call ahead and ask to see a menu so you can plan ahead.

2.	*Never go hungry.* To a restaurant, that is. If you have a small protein shake—or a half cup of fat-free cottage cheese and a slice of fruit—before you go, you'll take the edge off your hunger. This will make healthier ordering easier. If you're ravenous, even the pork rinds start to look good.

3.	*Skip the before-dinner drink.* If there's a seating delay, they inevitably send you to the bar to wait. Bad move. Beer and cocktails are high-sugar, high-calorie beverages. What's even worse is that they stimulate appetite, making you feel hungrier than you actually are. So skip the cocktail, and while you're at it, send back the bread basket, too, which is nothing more than a cornucopia of bad carbs.

4.	*Order off the menu.* Waiters and cooks are there to cater to you. Any good restaurant will tailor dishes to your reasonable request. Don't be afraid to make special requests to ensure that your meal is compatible with the Lean Body plan. Be explicit when you order your food: no added butter or oil, and only broiled, grilled, or steamed. Avoid red meats, gravies, and sauces.

5.	*You can have dessert . . .* just so long as you stick with a Lean Body–friendly dessert, such as frozen yogurt or sorbet. Always ask for fresh fruit on top. Coffee is fine, too, with a splash of milk.

Now, let's say you're faced with hard choices at a particular type of restaurant. For instance, you're at . . .

. . . an old-fashioned diner?

Ask for scrambled egg whites or an Egg Beaters omelet. Request that it be cooked in a nonstick pan with no grease or oil. Add onions, vegetables, or bell peppers, and top it off with salsa. Pair with a bowl of oatmeal with cinnamon on top, or a dry English muffin, and some fresh fruit.

. . . a Chinese restaurant?

Ask for your food to be steamed. Stick with chicken, shrimp, or scallops, and pair with steamed rice and Chinese vegetables. Make sure the food is prepared without MSG, which can give you an allergic reaction or force your body to retain more water than it should. Tempted to order an egg roll? Order a spring roll instead, which is usually chicken and vegetable wrapped in rice paper and steamed.

. . . a Continental restaurant?

Order grilled chicken or fish with spices on top, steamed veggies, and a baked potato or white rice.

. . . Italian restaurant?

Forget what Billy Joel said about a "bottle of red, bottle of white." Instead of wine, order a bowl of minestrone as an appetizer. For your main course, go for grilled fish. If you're having pasta, order a loose serving the size of your first—it's very dense in calories. Ask the friendly gentleman in the tux to add no butter or oil, and bring the marinara sauce on the side, so you can add it on your own. Same goes with olive oil; never let them cook your food in it. And as for dessert, let me give you the opposite of the advice in *The Godfather*: "Take the gun, leave the cannoli."

. . . a Mexican cantina?

Order grilled chicken or fish, but request that it be cooked without butter or oil. Also, order items made with corn tortillas, which are much lower in fat than flour tortillas. You can use all of the salsa, pico de gallo, and salad you can handle. Skip the fried corn chips in a basket; they're usually swimming in oil. If the restaurant offers baked chips, go for it, as long as you don't go *loco* with them.

. . . a seafood shack?

Fish is a healthy diner's best friend. Just choose one of the Lean Body–friendly fish on pages 65–66, and ask the waiter to have it baked or broiled with lemon instead of oil. Crab claws and lobster tail are fine, just so long as you don't dip them in white wine or butter sauces. Use red cocktail sauce instead. Even better, ask for cold lobster meat on a salad, then top with lemon juice or balsamic vinegar and a little olive oil.

. . . a steakhouse?

It may sound like heresy, but don't order a steak. Treat yourself to a grilled lobster tail or grilled fish. If you insist on red meat, order sirloin—one of the leaner cuts—and keep it to six ounces. Don't order "prime" or any of the rich, marbled stuff. Beef is typically higher in fat, and on this meal plan, the less you consume, the better.

How to Eat Fast Food Without Looking Super-Sized

The last thing you probably expected me to tell you is how to order at a fast-food drive-thru. But I'm a realist. When time is of the essence, and you forgot to plan ahead, I'd rather you make a pit stop at McDonald's than skip a meal. You just have to know the smart way to yell at that crackling speakerbox.

Some fast-food chains make it easier for you—with all of the bad press about overweight Americans and fast-food restaurants, the chains have responded with a line of healthier choices. But even if your favorite burger pit doesn't have one, you can still often choose items that are low in fat and lower in sugar and refined carbohydrates. Here's how.

McDONALD'S	Want a real happy meal? Choose a Grilled Chicken Salad Deluxe, which has 21 grams of protein with only 7 grams of carbs and a measly 2 grams of fat. Skip the dressing.
BURGER KING	Thank goodness you can order it "your way." I'd encourage you to go for the Broiler Chicken Salad with low-fat dressing, which has 21 grams of protein, only 7 grams of carbs, and 10 grams of fat.

WENDY'S   Wendy's was one of the first fast-food chains to offer a baked potato, which, paired with a chicken salad with low-fat dressing, makes for a lean meal on the go. You might also try the Grilled Chicken Sandwich, with 24 grams of protein, 36 grams of carbs, and only 7 grams of fat.

TACO BELL   Taco Bell is a good choice because they offer smaller serving sizes, which means you can snack a bit to hold you over until your next meal. Try the Chicken Fiesta Burrito, with 18 grams of protein, 48 grams of carbs, and 12 grams of fat. It's not perfect, but with only 29 percent of its calories coming from fat, it won't set you back too far on your Lean Body program. Or take advantage of the fiber content in Taco Bell food and order some Pintos and Cheese—with 10 grams of protein, 20 grams of carbs, 7 grams of fat, and 12 grams of fiber—which packs more fiber than anything else in the fast-food universe.

KFC   If you order a chicken breast and remove the skin, you'll be left with 29 grams of protein, with only 3 grams of fat and zero carbs. Make up for those carbs with a side order of BBQ Baked beans, which has 46 grams of them, and only 1 gram of fat. Add a piece of corn or an order of green beans, and you've got a meal that could even help the Colonel stay slim.

SUBWAY   That kid Jared knows what he's talking about. Try the six-inch Roasted Chicken Breast on Wheat, which has 23 grams of protein, with 47 grams of carbs and only 5 grams of fat.

CHICK-FIL-A   Surprisingly, that shopping mall favorite, Chick-Fil-A, boasts the sandwich with the lowest fat in our survey. Ask for a Chargrilled Chicken Sandwich with no butter, for 26 grams of protein, 28 grams of carbs, and only 3 grams of fat. (If you go for the fully loaded version with butter, that boosts the fat count to 7 grams.) Pair it with a side salad and a diet soda.

PART FIVE

The Workout

N ow here's the stuff you've been expecting, right? Dozens of pages that are jam-packed with iron-pumping, bicep-flexing, sweat-popping workouts? The kind of intense, take-no-prisoners fitness regimen you'd expect from a former Mr. Universe?

Guess what: it's not going to be anywhere near as tough as you might imagine.

My workout program has two simple components: the *Lean Body Power Workout* and the *Lean Body Cardio Workout*. These work together in a balanced way to strengthen your heart and lungs, burn body fat, and, most important, build muscle. They're the second part of the Banex concept of balanced nutrition and exercise. Exercise must also be balanced to get the best results in terms of health, energy, and body composition.

Why muscle, if you're trying to get lean? Muscle is the most metabolically intensive tissue in the body, yet conventional exercise programs ignore that fact. By performing simple resistance exercises—that is, weight training—you'll kick your metabolism into an even higher gear, enabling you to melt fat even while you're resting. In just 30 minutes per day, you'll be able to build a stronger, leaner you.

Cardio exercise, such as bicycling and jogging, plays an important role in the Lean Body program. Cardio burns calories, but, more important, it builds cardiovascular strength. In the Lean Body Cardio Workout you'll learn how to build heart and lung power and internal strength, all with a minimal investment of time. Say good-bye to endless, monotonous cardio exercises. I'll put it all together in a day-by-day format that will help you derive maximum results from a short workout.

In this part, I will unlock the secrets of body-transforming techniques for you and present them in a manner that's easy for you to use. The Lean Body Promise is the very essence of what I've found to actually work in getting countless others into shape. It *will* work for you. In as little as 12 weeks, you will see dramatic results and build exercise and nutrition habits that you can use for a lifetime.

What, Me Pump Iron?

You've got a bunch of misconceptions spinning around in there, and they've kept you from seeing the truth. Let me see if I can dispel a few of them for you.

Misconception #1: I don't have time to exercise.

Nobody has time to exercise. We live in the Age of Activity, where the idea of leisurely afternoons on the back porch have fallen victim to time-management courses and multitasking. And that's just before breakfast.

But if you think about it, exercise actually *creates* time, because it adds longevity. If you invest 30 minutes in yourself each day, you can keep yourself full of energy well into your golden years. You'll never have to deal with low energy levels, and you may even be able to avoid diseases that come with advancing age. Diet and exercise are the closest things we have to the Fountain of Youth. In the 30-minute daily sessions I recommend, you'll be set up with feel-good chemicals in your brain, energy, vitality . . . in short, waking hours that are more productive and enjoyable.

You have time for all of that, don't you?

Misconception #2: I'm fat because I was born with a slow metabolism.

Research shows that the majority of people have an average metabolism. But people assume they have awful metabolisms, because they see themselves gaining weight with ease. The truth is, if they were to start eating right and exercising, they'd see dramatic changes in their bodies.

Sure, there's a bell curve: There are some extremely skinny people who seem to be able to eat anything that's not nailed down and not gain an ounce. There are also morbidly obese people whose metabolisms work much more slowly than average. But no matter what, your situation can be helped. A clinically obese person may never be a waif-like model, but she can mitigate it—instead of weighing 300 pounds, she might be able to use diet and exercise to work her way down to 150 pounds—and keep it off.

That's because metabolisms—yours, mine, Ben Affleck's, Charlize Theron's—can be sped up. (Or slowed down, if you make the wrong choices.)

Misconception #3: If I work out, I'll look like a bodybuilder.

Hey, watch it!

Just kidding. I'm fully aware that you might not want to look like a professional bodybuilder. But you might consider this analogy: You probably don't want to be a NASCAR driver, either. But what if I said you had it within your reach to be able to drive like one? Likewise, what if I could show you a few simple techniques that champion bodybuilders use to achieve low body fat, boost their metabolisms, and, ultimately, shape their bodies?

A note to the ladies: I know the idea of getting bigger scares you. But relax; hormonally, you're not designed to build big muscles. This is a sllllowwwww process; you won't get big unless you purposely set out to do so. This program will, however, stimulate muscle tissue to help you burn fat more quickly.

Besides, muscle is more dense than fat. It takes up less room. In fact, five pounds of muscle is about half the volume of five pounds of fat. And muscle is what can give you those desirable curves (for the ladies) or brawn (for the guys). Muscle won't make you look weird; it will improve your appearance.

Misconception #4: Yeah, but I'm eating right. I don't need to exercise.

This is not true. Balanced nutrition and exercise (Banex) yields the best results. When following the Lean Body Meal Plan, you'll be in a *hypocaloric* state, which means you're running a slight deficit in the calorie department. When your body notices it's not receiving enough calories, it'll look for them someplace else. There are only two places: your fat stores or your muscles. Unfortunately, it's easier for your body to grab muscle and tear it down. And that's why a lot of diets fail in the long term: People cut calories indiscriminately, the body dips into muscle stores, and metabolism decreases. Which makes dieting all that more difficult.

But if you're exercising every day, your body will pause before breaking down muscle. Your body will think: *Hey, I need these muscles! I'm being stressed with weights every day! Guess I'll have to dig up those needed calories from the fat stores.* That's the unconscious, evolutionary thought process of your body. Exercising, along with a smart meal plan, means you can be in a hypocaloric state but keep your all-important muscles.

Misconception #5: I might exercise for a while, but then I'll say to hell with it.

Even if you haven't developed the habit of working out and eating correctly on a regular basis, you can reprogram yourself anytime to do so. Many of our daily habits are merely routine things that we do repetitively. Every morning we get up and we shower in the same way, dress in the same way, eat the same things for breakfast, take the same drive to work, shout "Yo, Big Guy" to Bob in Accounts Payable in the same tone of voice, and so on. If you think about it, your daily life is made up of dozens of routines.

I'm asking you to add just one more routine to your day: the exercise routine. Once you make the commitment to working out each day, no matter what, all you need to do is give it time. Maybe three or four weeks. The first couple of weeks may be tough. You might need to give yourself pep talks to get going. But by the third and fourth week, I guarantee that it'll be easier to stick to your program. By that time, you'll be noticing big changes in your body, and it will seem almost natural to work out every day. And by the end of the initial 12-week phase of this program, the exercise habit will become a part of your internal self.

Feeling Better About This Chapter?

These misconceptions are very familiar to me. I've heard many people say the same things during my years as a fitness expert and personal trainer to thousands. And all they do is hold people back from having the bodies they want.

Here's a quick preview: Exercising is only going to take up 2 percent of your time. And I'm going to tell you to take frequent breaks.

Still sound good? Keep reading.

THE SKINNY SO FAR . . .

▌ Building muscle will not only make you look great, but will also help you burn fat more quickly.

▌ You might think you don't have time for exercise, but you actually *create* time when you spend just a tiny portion of your week training your body.

▌ Balanced nutrition and exercise (Banex) are like the two wheels of a bicycle; try to use one without the other and you'll go nowhere fast.

▌ Give the program just one month. After that point, you'll have formed your exercise habit, which will make it easier to finish the whole Lean Body Promise.

The Two Kinds of Exercise

There are two basic types of exercise, and you're probably already familiar with one of them. **Aerobic** exercise includes activities like jogging, swimming, biking, and running from angry dogs. The word *aerobic* loosely translates into the idea that you're consuming as much air during exercise as your muscles need to perform that activity. That's why, if you're in decent shape, you can sustain a running pace for 20 to 30 minutes, or maybe even for the 26.2 miles of a marathon.

The other kind of exercise, **anaerobic**, is the opposite. Anaerobic exercises include activities such as weight lifting and chopping firewood, where your muscles are using more oxygen than your heart and lungs can pump into them. This is why you have to take frequent breaks to catch your breath, even if you're in the best shape in the world. Once your breathing stabilizes, the oxygen debt is cancelled. You're ready for more work.

The Lean Body Workout Program stresses a balance between **anaerobic** (aka weight training) and **aerobic** (aka cardio) training. If you want a leaner body, this method will give you the fastest results in the shortest amount of time. The weight training will stimulate your muscle tissue like no other exercise can, while the cardio will strengthen your heart and lungs.

Why Jogging Alone Doesn't Cut It

Cardio exercise contributes to favorable body changes. But it's easy to overdo it and sabotage your progress. Have you ever seen a slightly chubby aerobics instructor? Even though that person might be teaching a half dozen classes a day, doing hours upon hours of cardio work, they may be burning up muscle tissue right along with fat. As a result, the metabolism slows down. Enough slices of cake, and it's as if those hours of stair-stepping never happened.

Cardio is great for your heart, but so is resistance training. And unlike cardio, resistance training can kick your metabolism into high gear, helping you burn fat like there's no tomorrow. Cardio work alone just isn't enough.

There are benefits to aerobic training, which is why I want you to do cardio work in conjunction with your weightlifting work. Cardio work stimulates your heart and lungs, and does so for a sustained period of time, building up your lung capacity. It also gets your blood moving, which brings more nutrients and oxygen to your muscles, at the same time flushing away toxins and other metabolic nasties out of the tissue. (I like to think of it as a high-pressure wash for your muscles.) And of course, cardio helps burn fat, and every bit of help counts.

IT'S A MYTH:

"All you need is cardio—not weight training."

Cardio is all about burning calories, not stimulating muscle tissue. If you're not combining your cardio with a good resistance routine and nutrition program like the Lean Body Promise, chances are you're burning calories indiscriminately. (Those calories may be coming not just from glycogen and fat, but muscle tissue as well.) That's why you see a lot of what I call *skinny fatsos*—people who go to cardio classes religiously but fail to add muscle tone. Weight training stimulates all of the muscles in the body, so your body keeps them—after all, they're being used on a regular basis—and doesn't break them down for energy. Maintaining a balance of cardio and weight training is the key.

Resistance Isn't Futile

One of the world's foremost fitness researchers, Dr. Ronald Bahr of the National Institute of Occupational Health in Oslo, Norway, studied the effects of exercise on metabolism and fat burning, and came up with some really compelling stuff. Dr. Bahr found that intense exercise (resistance training) burns up more calories per minute, maintains muscle mass, and continues to burn up calories long after you've driven away from the gym.

Let's say you do resistance training for 30 minutes. Dr. Bahr's studies show that your metabolic rate will not only spike, but it will stay elevated over the next 12 hours. That means you could go home from the gym after work, have a snack, watch a DVD, then go to bed . . . and *still* be burning more calories.

Dr. Bahr also found that your body tends to use fat as fuel after an intense workout. During the workout, your body is using muscle glycogen (sugar stored in the muscles and liver) and circulating carbohydrates and some fat as an energy source. But after the workout, it kicks over and starts burning stores of fat. The study noted a 300 percent increase in fat burning after a session of intense exercise.

If you make resistance training—that is, lifting weights—the foundation of your exercise routine, and use the cardio stuff for support, you'll be building muscle. And building muscle revs up your metabolism. Consider this: *For every pound of muscle you build, you can burn 30 to 50 more calories per day.* A candy bar has about 250 calories. Pack on five pounds of muscle, and you can burn it off without even thinking about it.

Like Evolution, Only Quicker

When you exercise, your goal is to change your body. Your body is a biological organism that requires time to adapt to any new stimuli it experiences. Some are good; some are not so good. Give your body the wrong stimulus—for instance, funnel cake—and it will adapt (you will no longer fit into the tux you wore at the senior prom). Likewise, if you give your body the right stimulus—a Lean Body Workout—you can expect to enjoy certain adaptations. One is a sped-up metabolism.

The word *metabolism* is thrown around a lot; we discussed it back in Part Four in terms of your diet. There, you learned that metabolism is actually the sum total of all the calories you burn each day, both when you're active and when you're at rest.

What does a workout have to do with metabolism? In short, the more muscle tissue you carry on your body, and the more you stimulate that muscle tissue, the more your body will adapt, and the result will be a quicker metabolism. It's like evolution, only much faster, and on a more personal level.

Your Muscles Are Digital

've thrown around the words stimulus and adaptation. Now let's take a look at exactly what happens to your muscles when you put them through an intense workout (the stimulus), and how your body reacts (the adaptation).

I want you to flex your arm and pump your bicep.

Want to know what's happening inside your arm right now? If we took a cross section of your bicep muscle, it might look something like this:

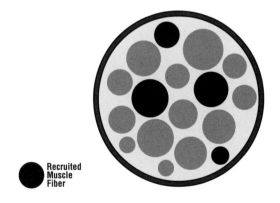

● Recruited
Muscle
Fiber

Cross Section of Muscle
Light Load on Muscle

Those little circles are your muscle fibers, and they're enabling you to flex your arm. Since you're not holding any weight, your body doesn't need to recruit many muscle fibers, maybe a handful. The rest of those slacker fibers are taking it easy, sippin' amino acids and glucose (sugar), and chillin' out.

Now pretend you're going to do the same flexing motion, but holding a 30-pound barbell in your hand. Take a cross section, and you'd see this:

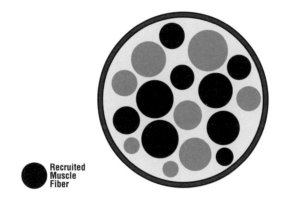

Recruited Muscle Fiber

Cross Section of Muscle
Heavy Load on Muscle

Since there's weight involved, your body has to recruit more muscle fibers. It can't just use the same few fibers and expect the job to get done. That's because muscle fibers contract according to the *all or nothing principle*. When stimulated, the individual fibers in a muscle either fully contract or do not contract at all.

If you're familiar with computers—or watched *The Matrix* once or twice—you know the basic concept of the digital world: zeroes and ones. It's the same thing with your muscle fibers: they're either resting (zero) or contracting (one). There's no 0.5, no fractions, just zeroes and ones.

The heavier the weight you use during an exercise, the more muscle fibers are initially recruited to enable you to lift that weight. Then, with each repetition of that exercise, those original fibers will tire out, and more will have to be recruited. This will continue until all available muscle fibers are recruited, contracting and eventually tiring out.

What does this mean for your resistance training workout?

Catch the Wave

Progressive resistance training is just a fancy term for lifting increasingly heavier weights over a succession of workouts. By gradually applying more—or different kinds of—stress to your muscles each time you work out, then allowing your body to compensate through the recovery process, your body will adapt by increasing muscle strength.

Say you're doing an arm curl with a weight, and you plan to do three sets, with 10 repetitions in each set. On the first set, your body might tap 40 to 50 percent of the fibers in your bicep to get the job done. After 10 of these curls, you'll reach a certain fatigue level.

Map this on a graph, it'd look something like this:

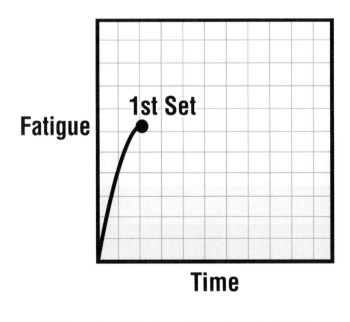

Fatigue in a Working Muscle: First Set

You've tired your muscle out to a certain point over a particular length of time, and now you're going to rest for about a minute. The fatigue level drops . . . but not all the way.

But don't rest for too long—just enough to catch your breath. This may be about a minute. Do another set of 10 curls, and your body will tap even more muscle fibers to get the job done—remember, those first fibers haven't completely recovered yet.

Now the graph looks like this:

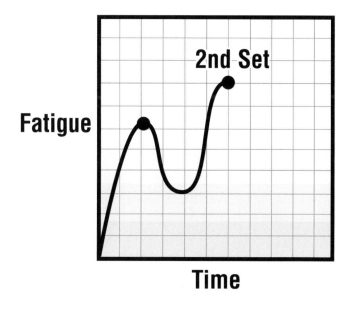

Fatigue in a Working Muscle: Second Set

Your muscles are getting tired now. Again, don't rest too long, and do another 10 curls. Now your body is thinking: *What? Those fibers are barely recovered from the first two assaults, and now I'm expected to lift more? I'd better tap even more fibers to appease this nut-case.*

More fibers are used, the fatigue level goes way up . . .

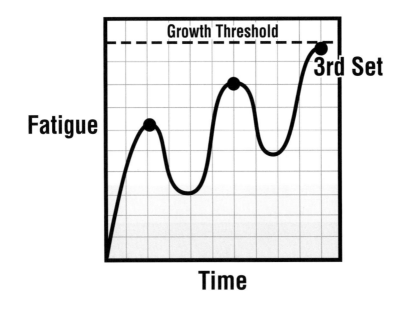

Fatigue in a Working Muscle: 3rd set

Congrats. Your body may not thank you right now, but you've reached the **growth threshold**, which is the singular goal of your weight training.

Enter the Threshold

The growth threshold is the point during your workout when the level of fatigue in the muscle is high enough that a growth response is sent to the brain, telling it that the muscle needs to adapt in order to accommodate future work. If your brain is a building contractor, and your muscle fibers are construction workers who have reached their limit, a growth response simply means that the contractor better throw some cash and benefits and extra stuff at those workers; otherwise, he's looking at a half-built office tower.

Likewise, your brain adapts by triggering muscle growth and increases in strength. How does this happen?

Whenever you lift weights, you actually cause microscopic tears in your muscles. Think of this as tearing down your muscles. With proper rest and eating habits, your body will quickly build those muscles back up, and they become even stronger than they were before. In the gym you tear down so that outside the gym you can build back up, better than ever. Remember the tagline from *The Six Million Dollar Man*? "We can re-build him . . . we have the technology." It's completely true. (And you won't need anything close to six million bucks.)

Your goal during a workout, then, should be to tire out your muscles as the workout progresses. You want your muscles to get increasingly tired until you reach the point where they are functionally worn out. At this point, any more sets or reps are a waste of time. The stimulus for change has already been sent. Mission accomplished. Take your ball and go home.

But it's not enough to merely exhaust those muscle fibers any old way. There's one other factor that will help you reach your growth threshold.

>> How to Recover

To maximize your body's ability to snap back from workouts, there are two things you need: plenty of rest, and the nutrients to repair the cellular damage you experience during workouts.

Shoot for seven to eight hours of uninterrupted sleep every night. During sleep, tissue is rebuilt and energy stores are replenished. It's normal to feel a little tired during the first few days when starting the Lean Body Promise exercise program. But if you continue to wake up tired after the first week, try increasing the amount of sleep that you're getting. Once your body gets acclimated to the program, you will feel more energetic, and you may actually be able to cut back a little on your sleep.

Eating all of your Lean Body Meals as detailed in Part Four will ensure that you are receiving all of the nutrients that your body needs to rebuild muscle tissue and burn unwanted body fat. Skipping meals will slow down your recovery time and will retard your results.

Intensity: The Key to Workout Success

Marathoners train by starting with shorter distances and eventually increase the duration of their runs. To build muscle, the opposite is needed: short, brief, heavy exercise—in short, intensity.

Intensity is the amount of work you perform in a given amount of time. To increase intensity, you increase the amount of work (exercise) or decrease the time (rest periods) or, ideally, both. Intensity is what determines how your body will respond to your workouts, because only through intensity will you reach the growth threshold.

Let's say you curl 50 pounds, 10 times. Then you go off and catch a movie. Two hours later, you'll probably be able to do 10 curls again. This is not intensity; this is just playing around. Your body doesn't have to adapt to anything. *Do 10 curls every couple of hours? No sweat. Already got it covered.* In other words, if you take too long a break, the muscle starts regaining too much of its original strength, and our goal through the exercise regimen is to get the muscle progressively more tired with each succeeding set.

But if you rest only a short period before doing that second set of curls, you might only be able to do eight. And the third time, maybe six. Your body is suddenly alarmed. *Wait a second—I've got much more work than I can handle. I'd better do something about it.* So it sends an adaptation signal to the brain.

How do you know if you're resting long enough between exercises, or resting too much? Let your body tell you. (Believe me, it will.) Once your breathing stabilizes, you've had enough rest. At first, this may take a few minutes, especially if you're out of shape. But eventually, you can condition yourself to keep that down to about a minute.

Here's a bonus: Because you will strive to keep your workouts more intense, they will be shorter. And that means you will not only get better results, but you will also spend less time in the gym. With the Lean Body program, you will eliminate wasted time and effort. We could all use some extra time, right?

THE SKINNY SO FAR . . .

- The Lean Body Promise workout is a combination of anaerobic (weight) training, along with some supplementary aerobic (cardio) training. Having a balance of the two is a key component of Banex (balanced nutrition and exercise).

- Cardio training alone can't give your body the muscle it needs to burn fat more quickly, nor can it give you the lean body you desire.

- The key to building muscle isn't the length of your workouts—it's how you push your muscles to their growth threshold in just three sets.

- It's also important to keep your workouts focused yet intense, which will trigger a response in your brain that will tell your muscles to grow . . . and fast!

Let's Get Started

Now it's time for a quick question: Are you 30 pounds or more overweight? And is your idea of an intense workout getting up from the couch to grab the remote plus making a quick dash to the kitchen for another can of beer?

Answer honestly; no one's judging you here. In fact, I admire you for the fact that you've picked up this book and have read this far; you clearly want to make positive changes in your life.

If your answer was yes, this next section is for you. This is an easy, catch-up program designed to coax you out of a sedentary lifestyle and into the right shape to begin the full-on Lean Body Workout Program, in just two short weeks.

If your answer was no, and you think you're ready to try the full-on 12-week program, skip ahead to page 119.

The Ramp-Up Program

Here's the plan: For the next two weeks, you're going to enjoy a "sampler buffet" of what's ahead in the following 12 weeks. Here is a list of nine exercises. (You'll find the full descriptions starting on page 130.) All you have to do is complete one set of each exercise—10 to 12 repetitions—pause to catch your breath, then hit the next one, and continue through the list:

1. Underhand Pull-Down (back, page 146)
2. Standing Barbell Curl (biceps, page 154)
3. Ab Crunches (abs, page 171)
4. Bench Press (chest, page 130)
5. Seated Barbell Press (shoulders, page 136)
6. Lying Barbell Triceps Extension (triceps, page 141)
7. Squat or Incline Leg Press (legs, quads, pages 159 and 160)
8. Leg Curls (legs, hamstrings, page 163)
9. Standing Calf Raise (calves, page 169)

The next day, skip the exercises and do 20 minutes of cardio work, either on a treadmill or stationary bike. The following day, return to the exercise circuit. The next, cardio. The next, circuit. (Do you sense a pattern here?) Do this for two weeks, and you'll be in fighting shape for the larger 12-week program.

The idea is to shake the cobwebs off your muscles and prepare them for the full program. No matter what shape you're in—or lack of shape—it's never too late to bounce back and reclaim ownership of your body.

Don't worry if you don't feel strong at first. Most people don't, so you're not alone. It doesn't matter whether you use 100 pounds or 10 pounds for an exercise. Your personal best is all that is required. The Lean Body Promise works for everybody and will work for you in the long run if you give it your best shot.

Your Simple Lean Body Workout Formula

Ready for the full 12-week program? Don't hit the gym just yet. It's important to walk in the front door with a battle plan.

I always say: If you fail to plan, you're planning to fail. That's why I want to make your planning as easy as possible. Start by planning your workouts on a monthly basis using the Monthly Workout Success Planner on pages 204–05. Then plan your daily workouts using the Daily Workout Success Planner on pages 198–99. Photocopy the chart, then take it with you to the gym and check off the exercises as you do them.

In the Lean Body program, I want you to do something every day—weight training or cardio. There's no day off. No need to groan—this program is designed to help you shed as much body fat as fast as possible. With only 30 minutes of exercise every day, you'll really be vaporizing that fat. (You won't be groaning when you drop a few dress or pant sizes, will you?) Think of the 30-minute daily workouts as only 210 minutes—only three and a half hours—out of your 168-hour week. It's important that you get used to the idea of daily activity as part of your life.

The Lean Body plan works on a three-day cycle:

Day 1: Weight training
Day 2: More weight training
Day 3: Cardio work

Then you simply repeat the cycle. If you have to take a day off, just pick up where you left off in the cycle.

Now let's get more specific.

The ABCs of the Workout

Workout A

Train the **push muscles**: in other words, first the chest, then the shoulders, and then the triceps. These muscles help you push weight *away* from your body.

Workout B

Train the **pull muscles**: that is, the back muscles and biceps, which are the muscles that help pull weight toward your body.

Workout C

Finally, we hit the **kick and crunch muscles**: legs, calves, and abdominals.

Need a visual? No problem. On the next page, you'll find a quick and easy guide to those major muscles, using my body during my competitive years as an example. (We used this photo because it's easier to see the muscles poking out!)

The order within each workout is important. For example, look at Workout A. During chest work, you're also using shoulders and triceps; during shoulder work, you're also using triceps. By the time you get to the triceps, they will be fairly tired, and it won't take much to stimulate them.

You may have noticed that there are two consecutive days of weight-training workouts, followed by a day of cardio, yet there are three separate weight-training workouts. That's because you'll be rotating the workouts over the training cycle as shown below. Here's how you're going to put this all together, with three sample cycles:

Day 1 (Monday)   A
Day 2 (Tuesday)   B
Day 3 (Wednesday) cardio

Day 4 (Thursday)   C
Day 5 (Friday)   A
Day 6 (Saturday)   cardio

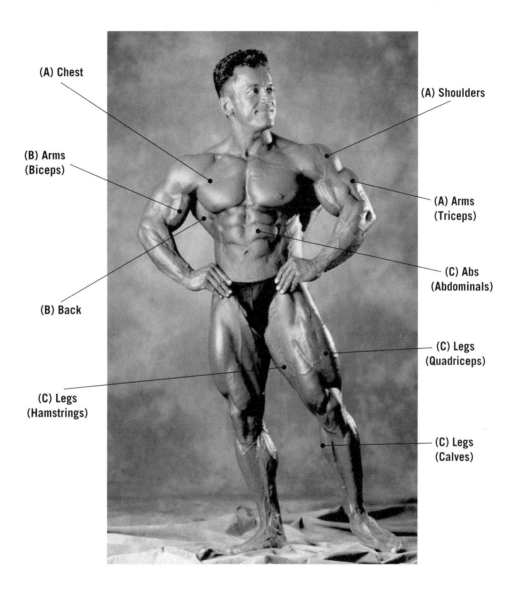

(A) Chest

(A) Shoulders

(B) Arms
(Biceps)

(A) Arms
(Triceps)

(C) Abs
(Abdominals)

(B) Back

(C) Legs
(Quadriceps)

(C) Legs
(Hamstrings)

(C) Legs
(Calves)

The Muscles and Their Corresponding Workouts

Day 7 (Sunday)	B
Day 8 (Monday)	C
Day 9 (Tuesday)	cardio

In short, you're alternating the weight routines every couple of days. This is great for a number of reasons. For one, you won't get bored with the same old three-day routine. (With the variety of exercises in the Lean Body training modules, you'll have enough variety to keep yourself—and your muscles—entertained for weeks.) Plus, you're giving your different muscles the time they need to recuperate. If you work your chest muscles on Monday, you're not going to be taxing them again until Friday, which means they'll have had four days to rest and adapt. Meanwhile, that cardio session you had on Wednesday will help get more nutrients to your chest muscles and flush out all of the toxins they've been storing up.

In many ways, this program is the best of both worlds: plenty of activity, and plenty of recuperation time.

The Three Essentials: Warming Up, Lifting, and Resting

Now you're ready for the three essentials of working out.

Before you perform your first set, you need to warm up. That's because your muscles are like rubber bands. When you exercise, you put tension on those rubber bands. The tendons—the tissue that attaches the muscle to the bone—are not as elastic as muscle. Tendon is like a nylon rope.

If your tendons and muscles are warmed up, they become more elastic and forgiving of loads imposed upon them. That's what we're trying to accomplish with a warm-up, which is especially important on those cold days. The idea is to heat up the muscles so they become less prone to injury.

So before the first set, take the first exercise on your list for that day, put on a much lighter weight than usual, pound through a set or two, and really wake those muscles up. You may even wish to warm up your body with five minutes of calisthenics or stationary bike exercise. *Now* you're ready for the tough stuff.

How to Lift: Stimulate, Don't Annihilate

The first part of lifting a weight is choosing it. You don't want something too light, otherwise you won't have a prayer in reaching your growth threshold. Likewise, you don't want something that will pin you to the floor of the gym.

The ideal is to select a weight you can lift about 10 times. And by the tenth time, it should be difficult to lift. Part of this is trial and error; you'll have to experiment to see how much you can handle. But here's the ideal lifting routine for each body part:

Each rep (that's muscle-speak for "repetition"—one single exercise movement) should take you one or two seconds to lift, and then two or three seconds to return to the starting position. The idea is to keep tension on the muscle at all times. Try to resist the urge to swing up and let momentum give you a hand. At the same time, don't let gravity help you bring the weight down. A handy rule of thumb: Pretend the weight is an infant. You wouldn't swing or throw a baby, would you? (Then again, you wouldn't bench press a baby, but let's not get into that.)

Quick Tip

If you really want to accelerate your fat burning, I strongly recommend doing some extra cardio. Workout B tends to be the easiest of the three, so add 30 minutes of treadmill or stationary bicycling after the weight training. That way, over a seven-day period, you'll have four cardio sessions instead of two. And you'll burn fat even faster.

Warm-Up

Two sets of the first exercise with a light weight. (This does not count as two sets of your workout.)

Exercise #1

Select a weight you can lift 10 times, then perform the exercise. This is your first set—muscle-speak for "a controlled series of repetitions." If this was too easy, increase the weight for the second set. Now perform the second set. Rest long enough to catch your breath, then on your third and final set, go for broke. Maybe you can do six reps, maybe more. But you should really work to tire that muscle and give your brain the stimulus it needs to order more strength.

Exercise #2

Repeat the process. (If you want to do one warm-up set, just for precaution's sake, go for it.) But this time, do as many repetitions as you can on the last two sets. After this exercise, you're done for that body part. It's time to go on to the next one.

>> Exercises That Should Be Outlawed

You might think that—to paraphrase Will Rogers—I never met an exercise I didn't like. This isn't true. There are two exercises in particular that I wish were against the law.

The first? Sit-ups. Everybody's been taught that sit-ups are good for your mid-section. But when your legs are straight, as they are in the traditional sit-up form, the main movers are your *psoas muscles*, a little-known group of muscles that run from the inside of the pelvic area to the small of the back. The psoas muscles do little for your waistline, and overworking them can stress your lower back. Want a simple way to turn this relatively useless exercise into a beneficial one? Bend your knees, which magically transforms a sit-up into a crunch. Then it becomes purely an abdominal exercise, with the psoas muscles and hip flexors out of the way.

The other exercise is called Good Mornings, where you take a barbell, rest it across your back, then bend over. It's probably earned the name because if you do it too much, you'll inevitably be shouting, "GOOD morning!" Well, stop your shouting. This exercise is extremely stressful on your lower back. Instead, try deadlifts and hyperextensions to give your lower back a proper workout. (See pages 151–53.)

Now you have only one or two more body parts to go, depending on the workout day. You're not trying to blow out your muscles here; you're exhausting them in a very controlled way. It's called *working the muscle to failure*—the point where you cannot perform any more unassisted work.

One quick note: Be careful with trying to work your legs to failure. Your body's survival instincts don't like it when your legs can no longer function—otherwise, how else are you supposed to walk out of the gym and make it to your next meal?

How to Rest: Quick Breathers

Rest long enough in between sets of exercises to catch your breath before you begin your next set. In general, you should rest about one minute between sets of smaller body parts like arms and abs; large muscle groups like the legs may require two minutes or more. Don't rest any longer than you have to, but let your body tell you when the oxygen debt has been cancelled and you're ready for more. That's when your breathing has normalized.

You might also pick up a simple stopwatch and set it for one minute. That way, you can train yourself to reach the ideal—a one-minute break between sets—before moving on to the next one. A chronograph with an alarm works just as well, too. These timers are especially handy if you meet someone in the gym who's chatty. "Whoops! There goes my timer! I'd love to hear more about your company's wild new spreadsheet program, but I need to be getting to my next set."

The break between exercises, by the way, should be however long it takes you to set up the machine/weights for the next exercise. The break between body parts can be three to five minutes.

Your Lean Body Exercise Menu

I've carefully selected exercises that can be done either with minimal gear in a home gym or on machines at any local or professional gym. Simply choose the body part you'll be working that day, select one exercise from the first module, another exercise from the second module, then go to work.

	Module 1	Module 2	Module 3
Workout A CHEST	Bench Press Dumbbell Bench Press Incline Bench Press	Flat Flys Pec Dec Incline Flys	
Workout A SHOULDERS	Seated Barbell Press Seated Dumbbell Press Machine Press	Dumbbell Side Laterals Bent-Over Side Laterals	
Workout A ARMS (TRICEPS)	Lying Barbell Triceps Extension Overhead Dumbbell Triceps Extension	Triceps Push-Down Dips Bench Dips	
Workout B BACK	Underhand Pull-Down Underhand Pull-Up	Bent-Over Barbell Row Bent-Over Dumbbell Row One-Arm Dumbbell Row	Hyperextension Dumbbell Deadlift Barbell Deadlift
Workout B ARMS (BICEPS)	Standing Barbell Curl Preacher Curl	Concentration Dumbbell Curl Alternate Dumbbell Curl Alternate Hammer Dumbbell Curl	
Workout C LEGS (QUADRICEPS)	Squat Incline Leg Press	Leg Extension Lunge with Dumbbells	
Workout C LEGS (HAMSTRINGS)	Leg Curls (machine) Leg Curls (lying with towel)	Straight Leg Dumbbell Deadlift Straight Leg Barbell Deadlift	
Workout C LEGS (CALVES)	Seated Calf Raise (machine) Seated Barbell Toe Raise	Standing Calf Raise Calf Press (on leg press machine)	
Workout C ABS	Ab Crunches Crunch Machine	Hanging Leg Raises Lying Leg Raises	

For example, if you're working your chest today, you might choose the dumbbell bench press from module 1, followed by the incline flys from module 2. The next time you work your chest (three days from now), you might choose the incline bench press from module 1, followed by the flat flys from module 2. The point is not allowing your body—or your mind—to become bored with the routine.

If you prefer to stay at home, purchase a 110-pound dumbbell set and a simple bench. The set doesn't have to be fancy and should run you no more than a couple hundred dollars. If you want, you can buy a set of Power Blocks (www.powerblocks.com) adjustable dumbbells.

But for about the same cost as setting up a home gym, you can join a local gym. Choose one that feels right to you. If you're not happy with one gym, visit another one. And another one, until you find the one you like best. Talk to the manager and get the lowdown—what the club is all about, what the clientele is like. Don't get pressured into signing an agreement for a gym that doesn't suit your needs. Every reputable gym will give you a free trial session before you sign up. Don't like it? Keep looking.

A NOTE ON SYMBOLS

 denotes an exercise that can be performed in the comfort of your home with minimal equipment, or at a professional gym

denotes an exercise that can be performed at any reputable professional gym

SAFETY COMES FIRST!

Before you try any of these exercises, make sure you have a clean bill of physical health from your doctor. (That goes double for back exercises, especially if you have a history of back ailments.) This is a program you will be pursuing on your own. There are no lifeguards on duty!

>> A Beginner's Guide to Getting Started

One of the reasons people get discouraged about their workouts is that they erroneously think more is better. "Great!" they exclaim. "I'm going to get into shape." The "Theme from *Rocky*" starts playing in their heads . . . and they end up getting sore or hurt—and eventually, they drop out of the gym for good.

Give your body a chance to adapt slowly—there's danger in doing too much too soon. There's too much of that "no pain, no gain" mentality in the fitness world. The idea is to challenge your muscles, forcing them to adapt—it shouldn't have to hurt. If your body is feeling sore and tired, your brain chemicals will be affected, and you won't be a happy person. And you'll be more likely to skip your next trip to the gym.

There are other things to watch out for. During the first couple of weight-training sessions—especially if you're not used to exercise—you might feel a little nauseous. That's normal; your muscles are probably kicking out a bunch of waste by-products. Or perhaps you ate your last meal too close to your workout. If you feel sick, or have cold sweats, or suddenly turn pale . . . listen to your body. It's time to stop. When you go back the next day, you'll find you can do a little more. Don't be discouraged. The toxins and by-products will clear out with every session, and those sick feelings will go away.

Bench Press 🏠

{A}

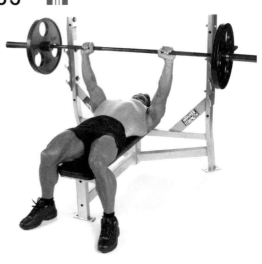

THE STARTING POINT This is probably the most familiar exercise here, aside from ab crunches. Simply lie on a workout bench with your feet flat on the floor. Grab the barbell using a shoulder-width grip, then lift it so that it's an arm's length away, and in line with your shoulders.

TIP I It helps to keep your head and hips on the bench, your chest held high, and your back slightly arched.

{B}

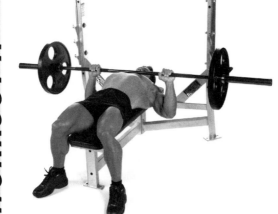

THE MOVE Lower the barbell to your chest (about even with your nipples). Your elbows should be kept back and your chest held high. Inhale as you lower; exhale as you push back up to the starting point. The idea is not to let the barbell fall to your chest, but for you to control the motion the entire time.

WORKOUT A ⟩ CHEST

Dumbbell Bench Press 🏠

{A}

THE STARTING POINT This is similar to the bench press, only using a pair of dumbbells. Lie on a workout bench with your feet flat on the floor. Hold a dumbbell in each hand just above your shoulders, with your palms facing your feet and your elbows out.

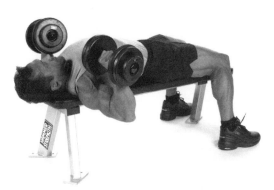

TIP | The path of the weights should follow in a straight line over your collarbone, not your face or belly.

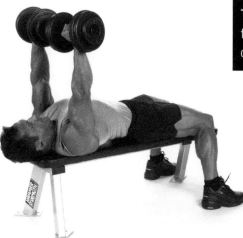

{B}

THE MOVE Press the weights up until your elbows are locked, then slowly lower the dumbbells back to your shoulders.

WORKOUT A ≫ CHEST

The Workout 131

Incline Bench Press

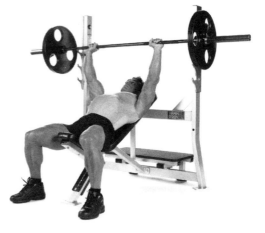

{A}

THE STARTING POINT Rest back on an incline bench. Take the bar off the rack using a grip that's about shoulder wide. Now you're ready.

TIP I When you lower the weight, aim for your upper chest; be careful not to hit your face or neck.

{B}

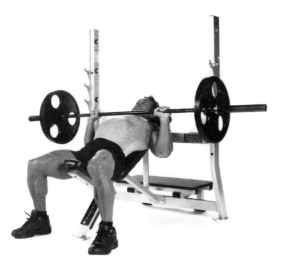

THE MOVE Inhale as you lower the bar down to your upper chest, then exhale as you return it to the starting point. Your head and hips should be on the bench, your chest held high, and your back slightly arched. As with the bench press, don't let gravity or momentum do the work: control the weight the entire time.

WORKOUT A 〉 CHEST

MODULE 2 Flat Flys 🏠

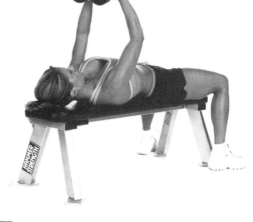

{A}

THE STARTING POINT Lie down on a workout bench with two dumbbells held above your head, at arm's length, touching each other. Your palms should face inward, and your elbows should be kept slightly bent throughout the exercise.

TIP | Don't lower the weights past the plane of your torso.

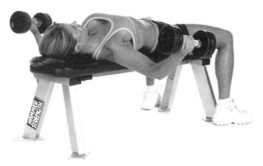

{B}

THE MOVE Inhale as you lower the dumbbells out to each side of your chest until they're about even with the sides of your chest. (Imagine making a semicircle pattern with both weights above your body.) Keep your chest high and your back slightly arched. Now return to the starting point above your body, exhaling as you do so.

MODULE 2 Pec Dec

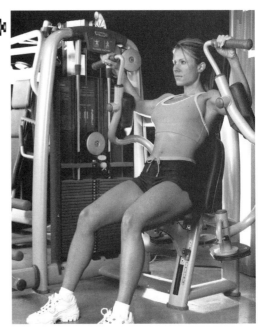

{A}

THE STARTING POINT This is essentially a fly movement, except it is performed in a vertical position, on a machine. Sit in the machine. Position your forearms against the pads. Grip the handles (if available) with your hands.

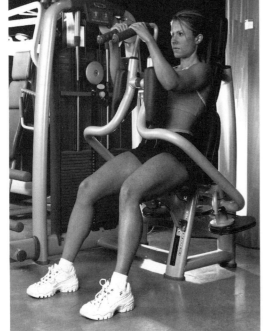

TIP | Push from your elbows, not with your hands. This will reduce the stress on your shoulder joints.

{B}

THE MOVE Inhale. Keeping your chest high and your back slightly arched, push against the pads with your forearms to bring the pads across your chest, or as close together as possible. Exhale, without letting your chest collapse. Repeat.

WORKOUT A > CHEST

MODULE 2 Incline Flys 🏠

{A}

THE STARTING POINT This is similar to the flat flys exercise, only using . . . that's right, an incline bench. What's the difference? Often a change of position can work your muscles in different ways; you want to always keep your muscles responding to a variety of demands. The incline bench throws the stress onto the muscles of your upper chest. To start, lie on an incline bench with two light dumbbells held above your head, at arm's length, touching each other. Your palms should face inward.

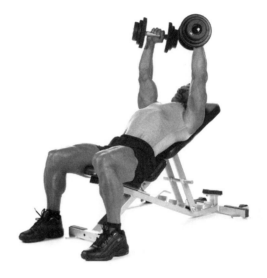

TIP | Keep your chest high, even as you exhale, to get a better contraction.

{B}

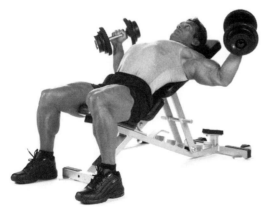

THE MOVE Inhale as you lower the dumbbells out to each side of your chest until they're about even with the sides of your chest. Keep your chest high and your back slightly arched. Now return to the starting point above your body, exhaling as you do so.

The Workout   135

Seated Barbell Press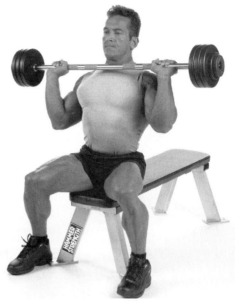

WORKOUT A ≫ SHOULDERS

{A}

THE STARTING POINT Here's a classic barbell press. Sit down gently on the end of a bench. Lift the barbell to your shoulders.

TIP I Keep your eyes on the barbell as you lift it overhead. This will help you stabilize the bar and keep you from hitting your head.

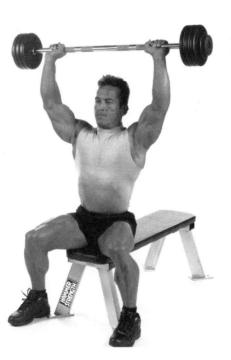

{B}

THE MOVE Inhale. Keeping your elbows in, press the barbell over your head. Your elbows should not quite lock at the top of the move. Now slowly lower the barbell back to your chest and let it rest there. Exhale as you lower the weight.

Seated Dumbbell Press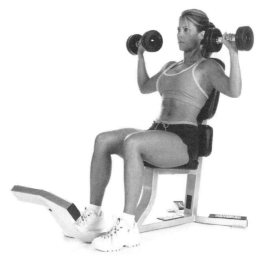

{A}

THE STARTING POINT Grab two dumbbells and sit on a workout bench. Lift the weights to your shoulders, palms facing inward. Make sure your feet are planted firmly, your chest is high, your head is up and your back straight.

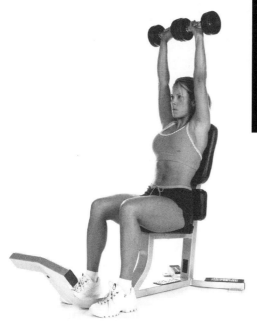

TIP | Rotate the dumbbells slightly as you lift them so that the heads of the dumbbells touch at the top of the movement. Rotate them back the other way as you lower so that your palms face each other again.

{B}

THE MOVE Keeping your elbows in, lift the dumbbells over your head to arm's length. Inhale before you lift, and then exhale as you lower the weights to their starting position.

WORKOUT A >> SHOULDERS

The Workout   137

Machine Press

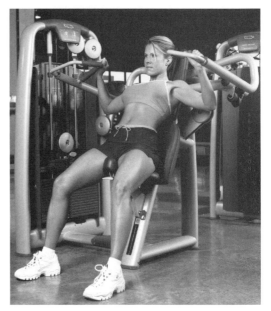

{A}

THE STARTING POINT Sit down on the machine press bench and grab the shoulder press bar. Your feet should be flat on the floor, your chest high and back straight.

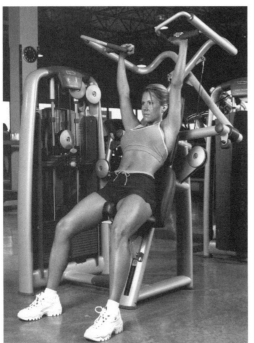

TIP | The key to using press machines is to use slow, controlled movements. Don't throw the bar forward like you're knocking over a stack of boxes; ease it out, then ease it back in. This controlled tension will double your results.

{B}

THE MOVE Inhale, then press the bar to arm's length. Exhale as you slowly return to the starting point.

WORKOUT A ›› SHOULDERS

MODULE 2 Dumbbell Side Laterals

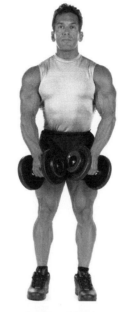

{A}

THE STARTING POINT Stand with your feet at shoulder's width apart. Grab two dumbbells and hold them in front of your thighs, with your palms facing inward and the dumbbells touching. Bend forward slightly at the waist, enough for the dumbbells to clear your thighs.

TIP | The dumbbells, at their peak, should be slightly higher than shoulder level. Turn your hands slightly so that the pinky of each hand is higher than the rest of the hand. Fight the tendency to let the dumbbells drop to the starting position.

{B}

THE MOVE Inhale, then bring the dumbbells up and out toward your sides in a controlled fashion. Inhale as you're lifting the weights, and exhale as you lower them slowly.

Bent-Over Side Laterals 🏠

{A}

THE STARTING POINT Sit on the end of a workout bench with your feet flat on the floor and your legs close together. Lean forward until your chest is touching your upper thighs. Grab two dumbbells and place them behind your legs, between your calves and the workout bench.

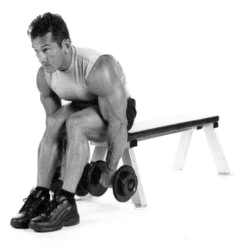

TIP | It helps to keep your arms slightly bent when performing this exercise. Turn your hands as you raise the dumbbells so that your pinkies are higher than the rest of your hands at the top.

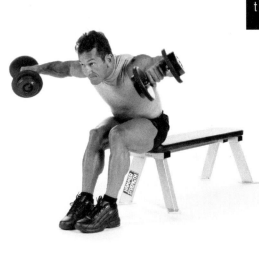

{B}

THE MOVE Inhale, then raise both dumbbells out to each side until your arms are parallel with the floor. Then slowly and steadily lower your arms back to the starting position. Don't lift your torso from the starting point, otherwise you'll be bringing in other muscles to help your shoulders. Let them do the work.

WORKOUT A > SHOULDERS

MODULE 1

Lying Barbell Triceps Extension 🏠

{A}

THE STARTING POINT Grab a barbell and lie down on a workout bench. Your hands should be about a foot apart on the bar. Press the barbell up to arm's length, straight over your shoulders.

TIP | If your forearms and biceps touch at the bottom of this exercise, you're doing it right. Be careful to lower slowly and in a controlled fashion so you don't accidentally hit your face.

{B}

THE MOVE Inhale, then lower the barbell to just above your forehead. Your elbows should remain pointed at the ceiling. Now press the barbell back to the starting point using the same arc of motion.

WORKOUT A ⟩ ARMS (TRICEPS)

MODULE 1 Overhead Dumbbell Triceps Extension

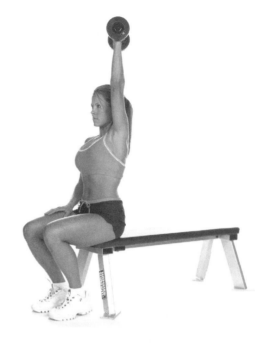

{A}

THE STARTING POINT Grab a dumbbell in one hand and lift it over your head. You may sit or stand for this exercise.

TIP | Be careful you don't drop the dumbbell on your neck or head.

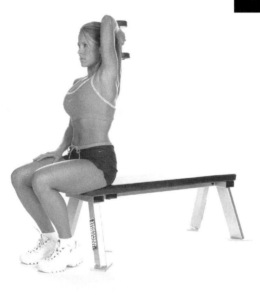

{B}

THE MOVE Inhale, then slowly lower the dumbbell back behind your head as far as you comfortably can. Then return to the starting point, exhaling as you do. You should keep your upper arms close to the sides of your head, and elbows pointed to the ceiling, as you perform this exercise.

WORKOUT A › ARMS (TRICEPS)

MODULE 2   Triceps Push-Down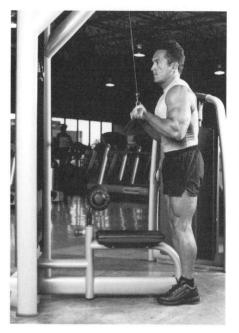

{A}

THE STARTING POINT   Stand in front of the push-down machine with your feet shoulder-width apart. Grab the bar with your hands about eight inches apart. Your palms should be facing down, and your forearms and biceps should be touching.

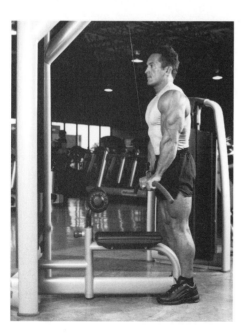

TIP | To really work those triceps, make sure your upper arms are planted at your sides during the entire exercise.

{B}

THE MOVE   Exhale as you push down in an arc to arm's length. Pause, then inhale as you follow the same arc back to the starting point. Keep tension on your triceps the entire time.

WORKOUT A » ARMS (TRICEPS)

The Workout   143

MODULE 2 Dips

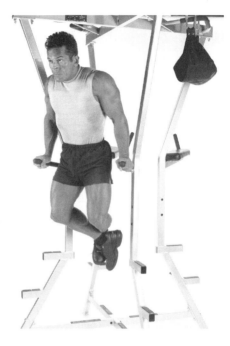

{A}

THE STARTING POINT Using a set of parallel bars, lift yourself up on the bars so you're held in place by your locked arms. Your feet shouldn't touch the floor as you do this. Bend your legs if you need to.

TIP | Try not to lean forward too far as you perform this exercise—you'll only make it more difficult for yourself. This exercise requires advanced upper body strength and should initially be attempted only under the supervision of a partner.

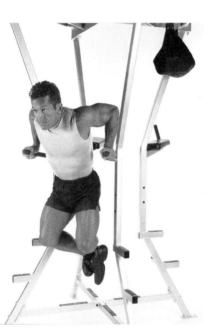

{B}

THE MOVE Inhale, then lower yourself down slowly while keeping your elbows at your sides as much as you can. Continue until you are comfortably stretched, then exhale as you press yourself back to the starting point.

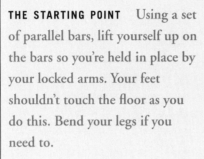

MODULE 2 Bench Dips 🏠

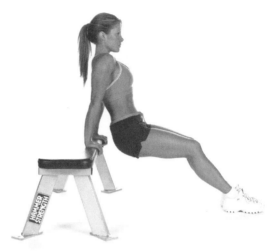

{A}

THE STARTING POINT Sit on the edge of a workout bench, with your hands gripping the edge of the bench at shoulder width. Place your feet together on the floor as far out as comfortable, then slide your backside off the bench, supporting your weight with your arms.

TIP I Make sure your hips stay relatively close to the bench, not out too far in front.

{B}

THE MOVE Keeping your elbows locked, lower your body until your upper arms are parallel to the floor. Then, push yourself back up to the starting point.

WORKOUT A > ARMS (TRICEPS)

On your back days, choose one exercise from each module for a total of three exercises.

MODULE 1 Underhand Pull-Down

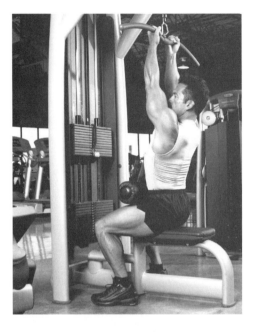

{A}

THE STARTING POINT Take a seat on the lat pull-down machine. Grasp the bar so your palms are facing you. Your hands should be about one foot apart. Your back should be arched slightly, and your chest held high.

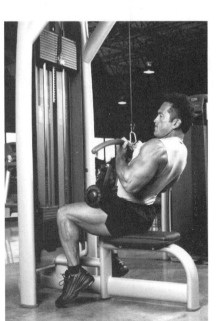

TIP I Pull your elbows down and back as far as you can, arch your back, and keep your chest out, as if you're trying to elbow someone behind you.

{B}

THE MOVE Pull the bar down until it is parallel with your shoulders. Inhale as you pull the bar, hold, then exhale as you slowly return the bar to the starting point.

MODULE 1 # Underhand Pull-Up 🏠

{A}

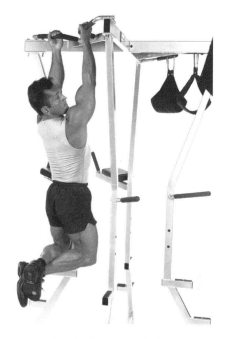

THE STARTING POINT Another classic exercise that all of us have tried at least once since we were eight years old and trying to impress our friends with our physical prowess. Grasp a chinning bar with a reverse grip (palms facing you) about a foot apart. That's the easy part.

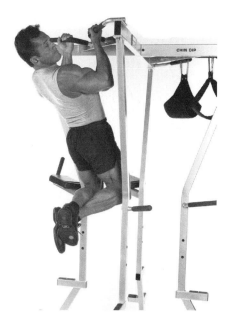

TIP I To maximize your back workout, arch your back slightly and lean back a bit as you lift yourself to the chinning bar. This exercise requires advanced upper body strength. If you're not there yet, use the underhand pull-down.

{B}

THE MOVE Inhale and pull yourself up. Pull as high as you can. Return to the starting point, but don't let your feet touch the ground. Exhale. Resist the urge to swing back and forth like a clapper inside a bell; you want to use steady, controlled movements.

WORKOUT B » BACK

The Workout 147

Bent-Over Barbell Row

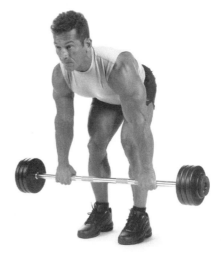

{A}

THE STARTING POINT   Stand in front of a barbell with your feet shoulder-width apart. Bend over and grasp the bar, making sure your back is parallel with the floor. Your head should be up, and your legs slightly bent.

TIP | Arching your back slightly and pulling your elbows back will help work your back muscles even more.

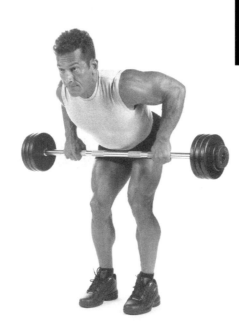

{B}

THE MOVE   Inhale as you pull the barbell up toward your lower chest, then exhale as you lower it. Do not let the barbell touch the floor until you've finished a complete set.

WORKOUT B ⟩ BACK

MODULE 2 Bent-Over Dumbbell Row

{A}

THE STARTING POINT Stand with your feet together and a dumbbell beside each foot. Now bend over and grab the dumbbells. Keep your legs slightly bent.

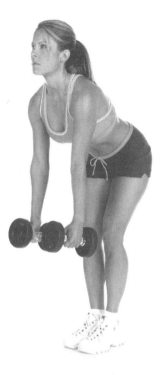

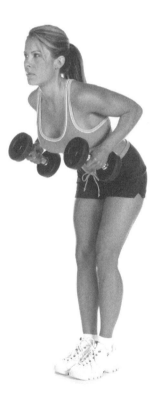

{B}

THE MOVE Inhale, and pull those weights up to the sides of your chest while keeping your back arched and head up. Exhale and lower them slowly to knee level. Don't let them touch the floor until you've finished the set.

The Workout

One-Arm Dumbbell Row

{A}

THE STARTING POINT Take a bench, then place a dumbbell next to it. Place one knee on the bench, keeping your knee bent at a 90-degree angle. Keep the other leg locked. Bend over and grab the dumbbell with the hand on the same side as the locked leg, using a "palms in" grip. Place your other hand on the bench and lock the elbow.

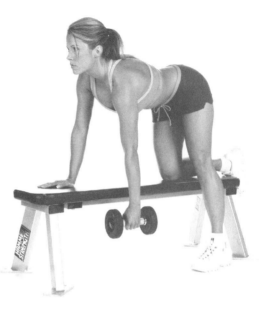

TIP | For maximum benefit, keep your working arm as close to your body as possible. Keep your chest out and back slightly arched.

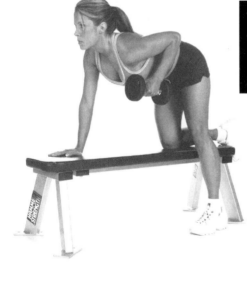

{B}

THE MOVE Inhale and pull your arm up and elbow back to bring the weight up to the side of your chest. Slowly lower the weight to the starting point and exhale.

WORKOUT B ▶ BACK

MODULE 3 # Hyperextension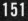

{A}

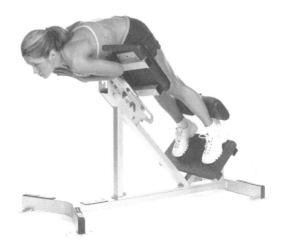

THE STARTING POINT Position yourself on the hyperextension bench so that your hips touch the end of the bench. Bend at the waist and face the floor. (You should look like the letter L.) Cross your arms and get ready for some fun.

TIP | Try to avoid swinging during this exercise. Keep your hips locked and focus on your lower back muscles.

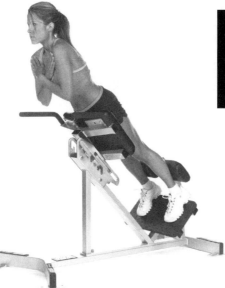

{B}

THE MOVE Inhale and raise yourself back up until your body is completely straight again. Slowly lower yourself back to the starting point and exhale.

WORKOUT B > BACK

MODULE 3 # Dumbbell Deadlift 🏠

{A}

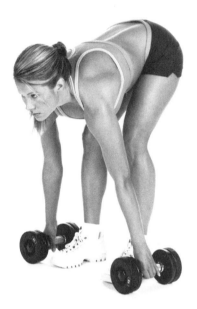

THE STARTING POINT   Place a dumbbell at each side of your feet. Stand with your feet about 10 inches apart. Bend at the waist and grab the weights, making sure your back is straight, your knees are slightly bent, and your head is up.

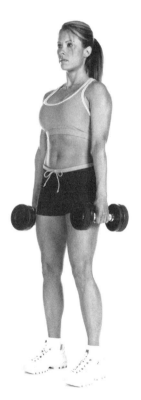

TIP I Keep the dumbbells as close to your body as possible. Focus on pushing your hips forward as you pick up the weights.

{B}

THE MOVE   Exhale as you stand back up with the dumbbells in your hands. Your elbows should be locked out. Lower the weights back to the starting point as you inhale.

Barbell Deadlift 🏠

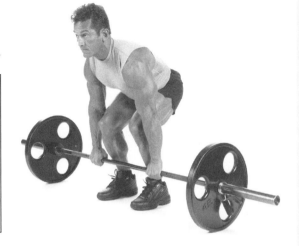

{A}

THE STARTING POINT Stand in front of the bar with your feet about shoulder-width apart. Bend your knees, bend over, and grip the barbell. Keep your back straight and head up.

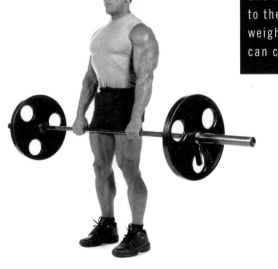

TIP I Remember to bend at the waist and knees as you lower the weight back to the starting point. Do not lower the weight with your legs locked out, as this can cause injury to your lower back.

{B}

THE MOVE Exhale as you slowly come up erect, keeping the bar as close to your legs as possible. Lower the bar back down slowly to the starting point.

WORKOUT B ⟩ BACK

The Workout 153

Standing Barbell Curl

WORKOUT B › ARMS (BICEPS)

{A}

THE STARTING POINT Stand, holding a barbell with your palms facing up. They should be about shoulder-width apart on the bar. The barbell should be held at arm's length, resting on your upper thighs.

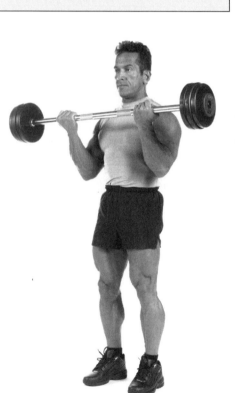

TIP | The trick is to lower the weight in a slow, controlled way; you want to make, those biceps work against gravity as much as possible. Don't let the weight just flop back down to your thighs.

{B}

THE MOVE Inhale, then curl the bar up to your shoulders. Keep your back straight, elbows at your sides, and your legs and hips locked in position. Then lower the barbell back to the starting point and exhale.

MODULE 1 Preacher Curl

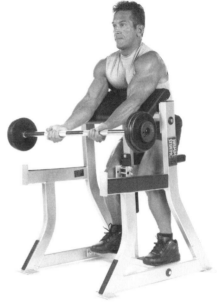

{A}

THE STARTING POINT   Sit at a flat preacher bench and grasp a barbell with both hands. Your palms should face up, and be about shoulder-width apart. The back of your upper arms will rest against the pad.

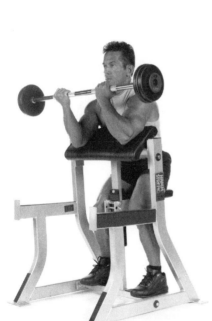

TIP | Resist the urge to move your upper arms outward during the exercise. Keeping them locked in place will make your biceps do the lion's share of the work. Don't let the bar fall into your shoulders at the top of the movement.

{B}

THE MOVE   Inhale and curl the weight up in an arc until it reaches your chin and your forearm and biceps touch. Then lower the weight along the same arc until you reach the starting point.

The Workout   155

MODULE 2
Concentration Dumbbell Curl 🏠

{A}

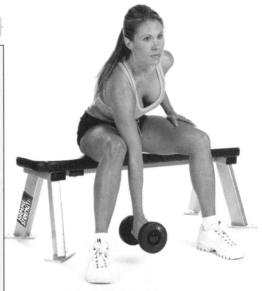

THE STARTING POINT Sit on a workout bench with a dumbbell in your right hand. Hold the dumbbell at arm's length between your legs. Place your left arm on your left thigh for support, then bend slightly at the waist. Finally, rest your upper right arm against your inner right thigh about four inches behind your knee. (You'll resemble a weight-lifting version of Rodin's *The Thinker*.)

TIP | Get a full contraction at the top by rotating your hand inward.

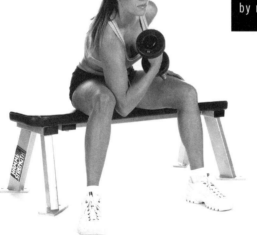

{B}

THE MOVE Inhale, then curl the dumbbell up in an arc until the dumbbell almost touches your shoulder. Follow the arc back to the starting point and exhale. Switch arms and repeat.

MODULE 2 Alternate Dumbbell Curl 🏠

{A}

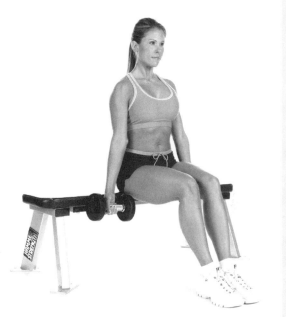

THE STARTING POINT Sit on a bench with a dumbbell in each hand. Make sure your back is straight, your head is up, and your feet are flat on the floor. The dumbbells should hang to your sides at arm's length.

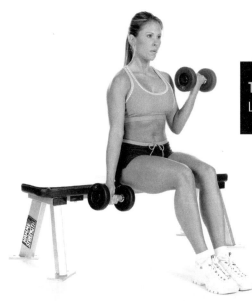

TIP I Keep your elbows at your sides. Lower slowly.

{B}

THE MOVE Inhale and curl the dumbbells alternately—right then left, right then left—keeping your palms up throughout the exercise.

WORKOUT B » ARMS (BICEPS)

The Workout 157

MODULE 2
Alternate Hammer Dumbbell Curl

{A}

THE STARTING POINT Sit on a bench with a dumbbell in each hand. Make sure your back is straight and your head is up. The dumbbells should hang to your sides at arm's length, palms facing inward.

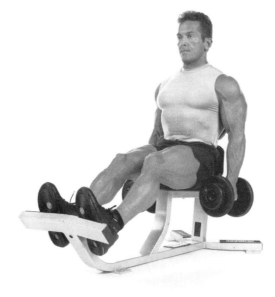

TIP | Lower slowly.

{B}

THE MOVE Inhale and curl the dumbbells alternately—right then left, right then left . . . *Wait a minute*, you might be thinking, *didn't I do this already?* Not quite. This time, keep the face of the dumbbell faceup throughout the exercise. It should look like you're holding a hammer (hence the name).

MODULE 1 Squat 🏠

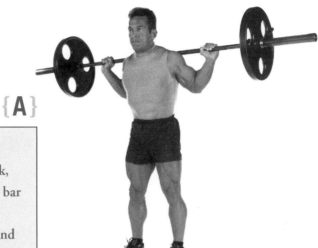

{A}

THE STARTING POINT Rest a barbell across your upper back, with your hands gripping the bar to help balance it. Your head should be up, back straight, and your feet about shoulder-width apart.

TIP I Resist the urge to bounce at the bottom of this exercise, which can strain your knees too much. Do not lean forward, as this can injure your back.

{B}

THE MOVE Inhale, then squat down slowly until your upper thighs are parallel with the floor. Keep your head up and back straight for the entire motion. Stand up again and exhale.

WORKOUT C ▸ LEGS (QUADRICEPS)

Incline Leg Press ⚏

{A}

THE STARTING POINT Lie back on the support pad under an incline leg press machine. Your feet should be 12 inches apart and planted firmly on the pad. Press the weights up until your knees lock. Release the safety stops, then grasp the seat with your hands underneath your buttocks.

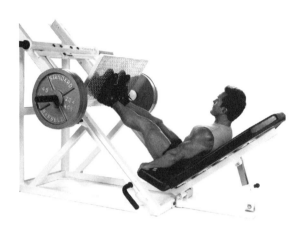

TIP I Do not lock your knees at the top of the movement. Maintain a continuous pumping motion and tension on your legs for the entire set.

{B}

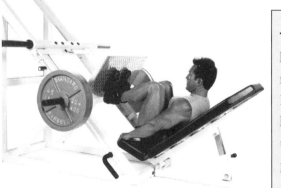

THE MOVE Inhale, then slowly lower the weight until your legs form less than a 90-degree angle. Keep your hips down and do not let your back or hips rotate upward. Push back to the starting point and exhale.

WORKOUT C > LEGS (QUADRICEPS)

MODULE 2 Leg Extension

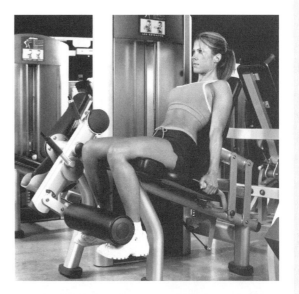

{A}

THE STARTING POINT Sit on a leg extension machine and hook your ankles and feet under the lower foot pads. Slide back until the end of the seat rests against the backs of your knees. Grip the sides of the bench just behind your buttocks. Point your toes straight ahead.

TIP I Keep your buttocks on the seat throughout the exercise.

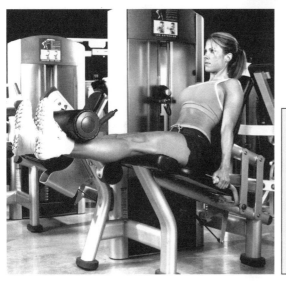

{B}

THE MOVE Inhale and raise the weights until your legs are completely extended. Slowly return to the starting point—don't just let gravity take over—and exhale. You should sit up straight and keep that position fixed during the exercise.

WORKOUT C ＞ LEGS (QUADRICEPS)

The Workout 161

MODULE 2 Lunge with Dumbbells 🏠

{A}

THE STARTING POINT Standing, hold two dumbbells at your sides with your palms facing in. Your head should be up, your back straight, and your feet planted twelve inches apart.

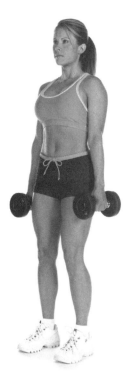

TIP I To lessen the strain on your knees, make sure they travel in line over your foot. Feel the stretch in your buttocks and hamstrings.

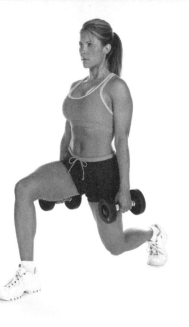

{B}

THE MOVE Inhale, then step forward with your right foot one stride, lowering until your right thigh is parallel with the floor. Meanwhile, keep your left leg behind you, not bending your knee until it is a few inches from the floor. Return to the starting point, then exhale. After you've worked your right leg, switch to the left.

MODULE 1 Leg Curls (machine)

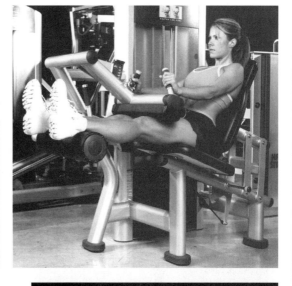

{A}

THE STARTING POINT Sit down on a leg curl machine. Hook your heels over the top foot pads, then hold on to the machine for support. Keep your back slightly arched, and your head up.

TIP | Keep continuous tension on your hamstrings.

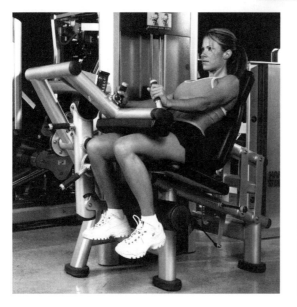

{B}

THE MOVE Inhale and curl your legs down as far as you can. Slowly return up to the starting point and exhale.

Leg Curls (lying with towel) 🏠

{A}

THE STARTING POINT Lie face down on an exercise bench. Then, have a training buddy place a towel across your ankles.

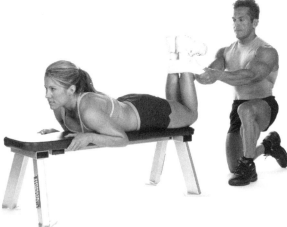

TIP I Keep your head and shoulders up during this exercise.

{B}

THE MOVE Have your partner keep constant tension on the towel as you slowly raise and lower your lower legs.

WORKOUT C > LEGS (HAMSTRINGS)

MODULE 2 Straight Leg Dumbbell Deadlift

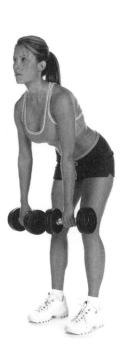

{A}

THE STARTING POINT Stand up with your feet a foot apart, then place a dumbbell at the side of each foot.

TIP | This exercise is different from the deadlift you perform for your back in that the knees are kept locked and you pivot at the hips, using your hamstrings to bring your torso erect.

{B}

THE MOVE Bend at the waist and grab the dumbbells, making sure your legs are locked at the knees and your back is straight. Keep your head up. Exhale as you stand up, keeping your arms locked out. Lower the dumbbells back to just below your knees—keeping your legs straight—and exhale.

MODULE 2 Straight Leg Barbell Deadlift

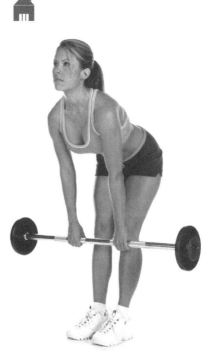

{A}

THE STARTING POINT Place a barbell on the floor in front of you.

TIP | While performing this exercise, you should think of pivoting at the hips, not the lower back.

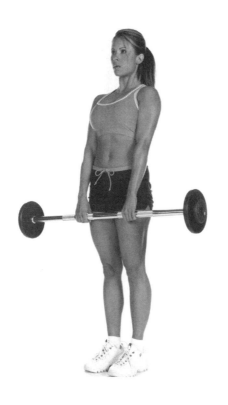

{B}

THE MOVE Bend at the waist and pick the barbell up with both hands. Keeping your legs locked, back straight, and head up, lower the barbell to just below your knees, or when you feel tension in your hamstrings. Stand erect, exhaling as you do. Repeat.

MODULE 1 Seated Calf 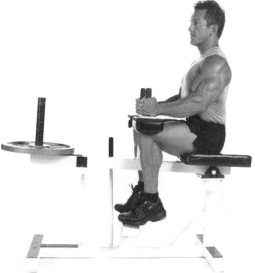 Raise (machine)

{A}

THE STARTING POINT Sit in a seated calf machine and place your upper thighs, just above the knee, under the pad. Put the balls of your feet on the foot rest. Raise up on your toes, then release the safety stops.

TIP | Avoid bouncing at the bottom of this movement, as it can cause injury.

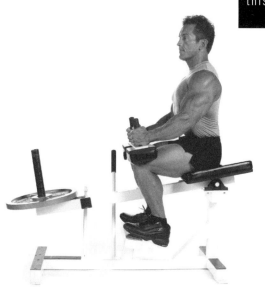

{B}

THE MOVE Lower your heels to the lowest possible comfortable position for a stretch, then raise up on your toes as high as you can. Hold this position for two seconds before you slowly lower to the starting point.

This exercise can also be done at home with a barbell.

MODULE 1 # Seated Barbell 🏠 🏋️ Toe Raise

{A}

THE STARTING POINT Place a thick board on the floor at the end of a workout bench. Hold a barbell with both hands, palms down, resting the barbell on your upper thigh about three inches behind your knees. Rest the balls of your feet on the board.

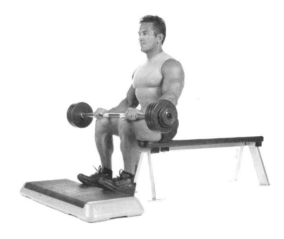

TIP | This, in effect, is the home version of the seated calf raise.

{B}

THE MOVE Keeping your back straight and your head up, raise up on your toes as high as you can. Hold this position for two seconds, then lower to the starting point for a stretch.

Standing Calf ✻ Raise

{A}

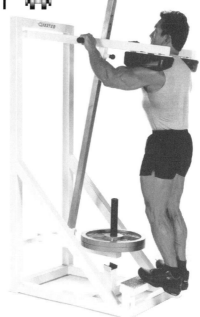

THE STARTING POINT Position your shoulders under the shoulder pads of the standing calf machine. Stand with your knees slightly bent, then place the balls of your feet on the foot pad. Rest your hands on the machine to stabilize yourself. Keep your back straight, head up, and knees slightly bent during the exercise.

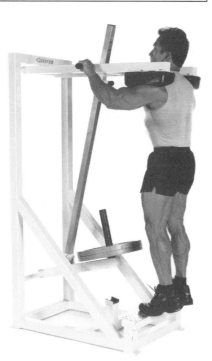

TIP I Keep your legs in the same locked position (with knees bent) throughout the exercise. Movement should be at the feet only.

{B}

THE MOVE Lower your heels to the lowest possible comfortable position for a stretch, then raise up on your toes as high as possible. Hold this position for two seconds, then slowly return to the starting point.

WORKOUT C ≫ LEGS (CALVES)

MODULE 2 Calf Press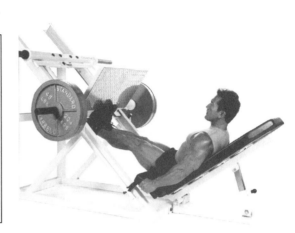
(on leg press machine)

{A}

THE STARTING POINT Lie on the support pad under an incline leg press machine. Place the balls of your feet on the foot pad, then press upward until your knees are straight and your legs are locked. Keep the safety stop in place with your hands.

TIP | Keep your hands on the safety stops so that they do not accidentally disengage.

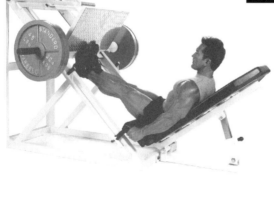

{B}

THE MOVE Press up with your toes, raising the weight rack as high as you can. Hold this position for two seconds and then slowly return to the starting point for a comfortable stretch.

MODULE 1   Ab Crunches

{A}

> **THE STARTING POINT**   Lie on the floor with your hands across your chest, your knees together, and your legs draped over a bench at an approximately 90-degree angle.

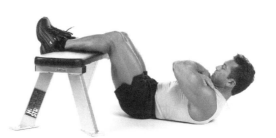

TIP | This exercise mimics the motion of rolling up a carpet.

{B}

> **THE MOVE**   Exhale and roll your sternum toward your pelvis, keeping your hips and knees locked in place. Hold this position and squeeze your abs once, then slowly lower yourself back to the starting point.

WORKOUT C > ABS (ABDOMINALS)

The Workout   171

Crunch Machine

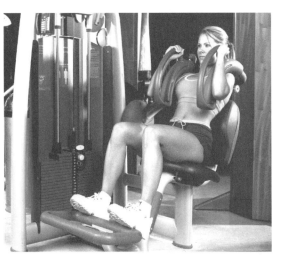

{A}

THE STARTING POINT   Sit in a crunch machine. Place your feet behind the foot pads. Grasp the bars beside your head.

TIP | Think of pulling your torso and knees together. Don't pull with your arms any more than you have to.

{B}

THE MOVE   Exhale and roll your sternum toward your pelvis, squeezing your abs and torso together slowly. Exhale as you do. Inhale, and repeat.

MODULE 2 Hanging 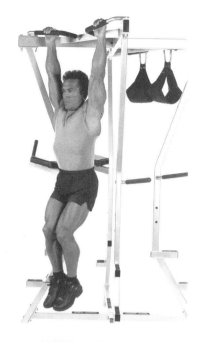 Leg Raises

{A}

THE STARTING POINT Stand on a bench and grab a chinning bar. (Your palms should face away from you.) Step off the bench and hang there, supporting your own weight with your arms.

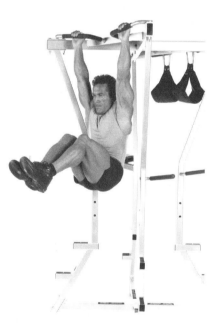

TIP I Keep your arms straight for the duration of this exercise. Think of your legs as providing resistance only. Focus on rolling your pelvis up and forward toward the bar.

{B}

THE MOVE With your legs bent at the knees, exhale and raise them until they are above parallel to the floor. Don't arch your back this time; keep it slightly rounded. Now slowly lower your legs back to the starting point and inhale.

WORKOUT C » ABS (ABDOMINALS)

The Workout 173

Lying Leg Raises 🏠

{A}

THE STARTING POINT Lie flat
on a workout bench so that
your buttocks are on the end of
the bench. Put your hands
beneath your buttocks, palms
down. Raise your legs until
your entire body is parallel
with the floor.

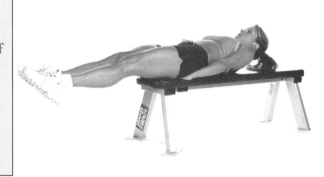

TIP | This movement will only work if
you roll your pelvis up and forward. Use
your legs only as resistance.

{B}

THE MOVE Inhale and bend
your knees, pulling your upper
thighs up into your midsection,
while raising your shoulders and
head to meet them. Round your
back, tilting your pelvis up as
you do this. Then slowly return
to the starting point (you as a
straight line) and exhale.

WORKOUT C › ABS (ABDOMINALS)

How to Do Cardio Right

In *Forrest Gump*, the title character loves to run. "That boy is a running fool," remarks one character as he watches Forrest speed by. He's got the "fool" part right. If you do cardio work willy-nilly, you may not get in shape as efficiently as you can.

Basically, there are two ways you can do cardio. You choose **LSD**—no, not the hallucinogenic, but "long, slow distance." Or, you can choose **HIT**—"high-intensity training." If you've got all the time in the world, LSD is fine for burning body fat. But if you want the greatest results in the shortest amount of time, my advice to you is to drop the LSD and instead HIT it. (Sorry. I've been waiting this entire book to make that joke.)

In other words, forget about wasting 45 minutes on a bike or treadmill doing long, slow distance. Instead, with HIT, you mix up high-intensity periods of aerobic training with low-intensity periods. Let's say you hop on an exercise bike with three kinds of resistance levels: easy, moderate, and difficult. Follow this 26-minute routine:

Minutes 1–2: Level one (easy)
Minutes 3–5: Level two (moderate)
Minutes 6–9: Level three (difficult)

In just under 10 minutes, you've upped the intensity to the highest level. Now you're going to ease back and allow your heart and lungs to slow down before going back up.

Minutes 10–11: Level two
Minutes 12–15: Level three

You're back up again in just five minutes. Now you're ready to ease back down again:

Minutes 16–17: Level two
Minutes 18–21: Level three
Minutes 22–24: Level two
Minutes 25–26: Level one

If you were to map this out, it would resemble a series of hills. And in fact, that's what you're doing—taking your bike up and down hills of various intensity. Why is this optimal? Because you're doing more to stimulate your metabolism, and the total effect is that you're burning more calories. And the effect lasts for hours afterward.

Take a look:

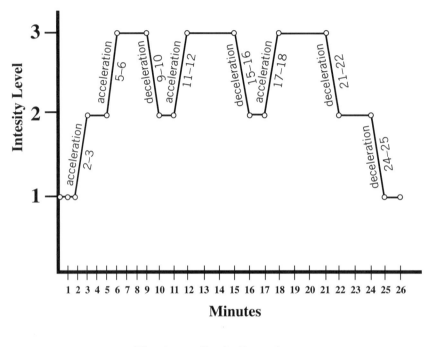

The Lean Body Promise
Cardio Workout Chart

You don't have to do this on a stationary bike. You can also simulate the three levels of intensity on a stair-climber machine, treadmill, or jogging track. Here are three additional pointers to keep in mind when you're doing cardio work:

1. *Keep your cardio sessions longer than 20 minutes but shorter than 45 minutes.* During the first 20 minutes of, say, jogging, your body is burning glucose and glycogen along with stored body fat for energy. But once you pass the 20-minute mark, your body gradually shifts over into burning stored fat. So if you want your cardio work to burn fat, you've got to reach beyond this time limit. At the same time, you don't want to go beyond 45 minutes, because then your body will start digging into your lean muscle stores for energy, using up amino acids required for muscle growth and recuperation. Lose the muscle and you lose your natural fat burner.

2. *Do it first thing in the morning.* If possible, it's best to perform cardio work after you've had a substantial fast. If you're like most people—that is, you haven't mounted a commando raid on your fridge in the middle of the night—you probably wake up without having eaten for six to eight hours. This is perfect. Pour yourself a cup of joe, slug it down, then hop on the treadmill or bike, or head outside for that run. If you can't do it first thing in the morning, make sure you hit it when you're getting hungry at some point during the day.

   If you absolutely must do cardio on the same day as your weight training, perform your cardio *after* your weight training. At that point, you'll have burned up your muscle glycogen (stored carbs) during weight training, and your body will be ready to switch over to burning stored fat.

3. *Put your heart into your exercise routine . . . but not all of it.* If you perform your cardio work too intensely, you'll push your body into the anaerobic range, which means you'll be burning glycogen, not fat. (And by the same token, if your intensity level is too low, you burn too few calories.) Ideally, your heart rate should be at about 75 to 85 percent of its maximum.

How do you figure out your optimal heart rate? The simplest way is to gauge by your breathing. If you're running out of breath, you're going too fast. By the same token, if you don't feel yourself working at all, consider upping the intensity.

Or you can try this simple formula: Take the number 180 and subtract your age. This is your ballpark target heart rate. For example, if you're 30 years old, your ideal heart rate is 150 beats per minute.

Now track your heart rate by placing your index finger on your carotid artery on the left side of your neck. Using a watch, or the clock on the gym wall, count the number of beats in a 15-second period. Multiply that by four, and presto. Your heart rate, in beats per minute. (If you count 30 beats in that 15-second period, that means you're working at 120 beats per minute.)

Some gym machines even have fingertip sensors that automatically calculate this for you. But once you know how your ideal heart rate feels, you'll be able to instantly judge your intensity level.

Baby Got (Feed)Back: The Easiest Way to Stay Motivated

Earlier in this book, you learned that you can build your motivation just as you do a muscle. By exercising your motivation daily, it will grow over time. Research shows that one of the key components of building personal motivation is experiencing positive feedback. We all know about positive feedback, don't we? From the first time our parents said "Good job!" when we learned a new skill, we felt the rush of a positive accomplishment.

In the Lean Body program, you can experience positive feedback in many ways: inches lost from your waist, hips, arms, and legs; or pounds of body fat lost; or shrinking dress or pant sizes.

But one of the best ways of receiving positive feedback is by using progress photos, those classic "before and after" shots. The difference is, you'll just start with a "before" shot, and continually check your progress against it. A before photo lets you know exactly what you look like now. It's the closest thing we have to being able to step outside our own bodies and take a look back. Videotape works well, also.

In order to be successful on your journey of transformation, you need to know your starting point. Taking a before photo might seem like an awkward thing to do, especially if you think you're really out of shape. But if you don't, how will you know how much progress you've made 12 weeks from now?

I promise you that if you take your picture and study it, you'll receive two things:

1. a record of what you look like now so you can measure progress and chalk up victories in the weeks to come, and

2. strong incentive to change. Many people look at their before pictures and mutter to themselves: *I'm tired of looking this way. I'm going to do something about it.*

Take your picture in comfortable-yet-shape-revealing clothes, such as a leotard (if you're female), gym shorts (if you're male), or a polka-dot inner tube and a feathered boa (if you're eccentric). A bathing suit works, too. Make sure you're holding a newspaper so that the date can be seen. You'll want to prove to your friends how quickly you burned fat and sculpted your body. Take a total of three pictures: one from the front, one from the back, and one from the side.

And don't forget to smile.

Rested Up?

Congrats—you're now well on your way to making the Lean Body Promise a reality in your own life. There's just one small additional step: putting everything you've learned together.

Once you've caught your breath from those Hanging Leg Raises—they're a bit challenging, aren't they?—turn the page for the final leg of your Lean Body journey.

PART SIX

Putting It All Together

I f this book were a Star Wars movie, you'd be ready for Jedi knighthood right about now. You've read the stories of other Jedi knights who started out just like you—eager individuals who were tired of the way they looked and wanted to break free of their negative lifestyle habits (Part Two). You've studied the mystical ways of human motivation (Part Three); the simple secrets of healthy nutrition (Part Four); and the most effective ways to shape your body into a lean, mean healthy machine.

Now, young Padawan Learner, you are ready for the final part of your Jedi training. No, it doesn't involve a light saber. (Though one would be handy for vaporizing all of the junk food in your house.) The final part of your training involves 10 simple steps to put it all together—to implement your Lean Body Promise. In this part, I'll show you how to use everything you've learned so far to make dramatic changes in your body.

Ready for the first step? You're already two-thirds of the way there.

Step #1: Make the Decision

The first step is the most important: making the conscious decision to change your life. Picking up a copy of this book was an important part of it, as was reading this far into the book. (I hope you haven't skipped to this section for the surprise twist at the end. If so, let me reveal it now: Darth Vader is Luke Skywalker's father.) Now all that's left is for you to say, "Yes, I'm going to give this a shot. A small slice of my time every day is nothing, compared to the lifetime benefits I can receive."

Still not convinced? Do me a favor and skip back to Part Two, where you can review stories of successful Lean Body Challengers. They succeeded against odds (debilitating illness, time constraints, paralysis) that may have been worse than the ones you face. So what's your excuse for not trying?

Step #2: Sign Your Name

Banks make you sign promissory notes. Lawyers make you sign agreements. Kids make you sign homework. Now I want you to make a written commitment to the Lean Body program for the next 12 weeks . . . and sign it.

On page 187 of this book, you'll find a commitment letter printed in full. Tear it out, or if you can't stand the thought of damaging this defenseless book, photocopy it. Or, you can access a printable form online at www.leanbodypromise.com. Read it, sign it, date it, then fax or mail it to me, personally, here at Labrada headquarters in Houston, Texas. Once I receive it, I'll sign you up for the free *Lean Body Coaching Club* e-newsletter that will provide you with tips and valuable info specific to your 12-week challenge.

Step #3: Clean Out Your Fridge

This is the fun part. I want you to clean out your fridge and cupboard, tossing anything that's not part of the Lean Body Meal Plan outlined in Part Four. (If you live with a spouse and children, or roommates, you'd better receive clearance first.) The point is to limit the distractions. It'll be far easier to stick to your healthy, nutritious meals if you're not staring at sugar-sweet, overprocessed foods every time you open a pantry cabinet.

You don't want to stare at empty shelves, either. That's why you should take the Lean Body Fridge List (Appendix G) and go to town. You don't have to find a fancy health food market; every ingredient in the Lean Body Meal Plan can be found at any good neighborhood supermarket.

Step #4: Prepare Your Home Gym, or Join One

Next, I want you to decide if you're going to work out at home or at a gym. Again, you shouldn't feel intimidated about walking into a commercial gym—these days, gyms cater to the everyday crowd more than they do gym rats and bodybuilders. Some people prefer a spartan, plain Jane, black iron weight gym, while other people aren't happy unless they're ensconced in a high-end mirrored spa with chrome machines and Kenny G, saxophone wailing in the background. Whatever works for you. Just don't forget you're there to work your body.

Step #5: Schedule It

O nce you find the gym of your dreams . . . make sure you go to it.

Sounds simple, right? It's not. Many people sign up with the best intentions, but then let their membership collect dust and spiderwebs. A gym membership is only good if you use it. You're giving them your hard-earned dough; why not go every day and get your money's worth?

The easiest way to make sure you hit the gym every day is to schedule your workouts. Use the Monthly Workout Success Planner on page 204 of this book. As you finish the workouts, you can take satisfaction in crossing those babies off.

Step #6: Do It

S teps one through five were all important "setup" steps. Now comes the moment of truth: actually *doing* the Lean Body program.

Don't let the moment overwhelm you. Don't rationalize putting it off. Just simply get started today.

Every successful Lean Body Challenger I've met has told me the same thing: you have to take the program day by day. Nobody bites off life in 12-week chunks; we're only human. We can only digest one day at a time. And that's all I'm asking.

Approach it on a day-to-day basis, and I promise you: before you know it, you'll be ready to . . .

Step #7: Savor the Results

A fter the 12-week challenge is over, take a moment to mail me your before and after photos, and a short line or two about the results you've achieved. After I admire your hard work, I'll send you a certificate of completion—let's face it, after 12 weeks of this program, you're probably going to want to show it off to friends. Also, your name will be added to the growing number of successful Lean Body Challengers at www.leanbodypromise.com.

But there's no certificate that can compare to your real prize: your new Lean Body. Enjoy it!

Step #8: Care and Maintenance of Your Lean Body

*O*kay, you might be thinking. *I've done it.*

I successfully completed the Lean Body Promise. Lost the body fat. Packed on the lean muscle. I feel more energetic than I ever have in my life, and I've never looked better. Members of the opposite sex smile at me. Dogs stop to lick my hand.

. . .

Yep, I did it.

. . .

Okay, then.

. . .

[Time passes.]

. . .

Yessirree, I did it.

. . .

Oh yeah.

. . .

Uh . . . Lee? What now?

This is a question I hear all of the time. What do I do after the 12-week challenge? Here I am, I've made some great changes, but I'm not finished. What do I do now?

Here's my answer: Stick with the diet and the exercise program, until you reach your desired goal. Once you're at your desired goal, you don't want to lose more body fat; it's time to maintain.

To maintain, you should increase your caloric intake by about 10 percent—which simply means you should eat a little more protein and carbohydrates. One of the things that sometimes happens when your body fat percentage starts to dip down toward the single digits is that you get hungry more often. So instead of your usual palms and fists at meals, go for a palm and a fist with an extra finger. (Sounds bizarre, I know, but work with me here.) Or even a fist and a half for the good carbs. You might also want to boost your intake of essential fats—some additional nuts, avocados, or olive or flaxseed oil.

By increasing your caloric intake a little bit—not going hog wild by adding "cheat weeks" to your nutrition plan—you should reach a point of **homeostasis**. This is where you're neither gaining nor losing, and you're not hungry. This is the status quo. Or as the philosopher Goldilocks once said, "Just right."

Step #9: Stay in Touch with Your Lean Body Coach

'll continue to be there for you, as your Lean Body Coach and mentor. As a reader of *The Lean Body Promise*, you have free access to up-to-the-minute information on training and nutrition. You can even ask questions and get answers to all of your questions. It's the year-round support you need to stay at your best. Just go to www.lean bodypromise.com and sign up for my free e-newsletter.

I can't wait to hear from you.

Step #10: Become a Fitness Evangelist

Now that you've gotten yourself in shape and you're enjoying this program, don't be selfish and keep it to yourself. Share it with other people. E-mail your friends and family the link to my website (www.leanbodypromise.com and www.leanbody coach.com). Also make it your goal to get out and turn other people on to this healthy program and book.

Why? A couple of reasons. Some of them are even downright selfish.

For one, the feeling of helping others can be extremely gratifying. If you can serve as an inspiration to others, you'll gather a group of people (call them your "fans") who look up to you for inspiration. Suddenly, you're more accountable, because guess what: you've become a role model. You don't want to let everyone else down.

But I'm also making an appeal to your altruistic side. (Come on, I know it's in there somewhere.) By doing this, you're helping to take a bite—pardon the pun—out of the chronic obesity epidemic in the United States. Think about the cascading effect: you're helping people become less obese, people who are going to be healthier and more productive. It's estimated that obesity costs us over $120 billion a year in health care costs right now. Somebody's got to pick up the tab for it—and it's usually us, paying higher insurance premiums and taxes.

There are many good reasons for all of us to help each other beat this obesity problem. Spread the word . . . starting with your own family. Then share this book with a neighbor or a friend. Be a fitness evangelist. Together we can change the world, one person at a time.

My Lean Body Promise Letter »

"There is a strong, lean body inside me, and I have the power to release it."

I am embarking on a life-changing journey that begins now, with my Lean Body Promise program. I am doing this for myself because I care enough about myself that I want to change. I want to improve my appearance, strength, self-image, and confidence.

It doesn't matter if I have failed to get into shape before; this is the only time that matters, and I will succeed. I am changing my old habits and replacing them with new ones.

I am going to build my body and my willpower. I have the power to improve myself and I am taking control.

I will faithfully stick with my Lean Body Promise program for the next 12 weeks. To that end, I make the personal commitment to:

- Build my willpower and motivation by getting rid of excuses. I will foster positive thoughts and get right back on track if I mess up, as discussed in the Lean Body Promise motivation section (Part Three).
- Plan and eat my meals as recommended in the Lean Body Promise nutrition program (Part Four).
- Plan my workouts, and exercise when I am scheduled to, as demonstrated in the Lean Body Promise workout (Part Five).

Sincerely,

Your Signature Here _____

Printed Name _____

E-mail Address _____

Mailing Address _____

City, State, ZIP _____

Note: this form is meant to be filled out and sent in to Lee for accountability.

Please send it to the attention of Lee Labrada:

E-mail it   leanbodypromise@labrada.com

Fax it   1-281-209-2135

Mail it   P.O. Box 62436
           Houston, TX 77205

PART SEVEN

Lean Body FAQs

MMMMrrphhfff. Wazzat? Oh, no. (Tastes inside of mouth.) I slept through the alarm again. I'm going to be late for work. Nuts. I should just skip breakfast, shouldn't I?

No. Breakfast is the most important meal of the day. You need to get food into your body and—as the name implies—"break the fast." Your body is starving for two things: amino acids from protein, and enough energy to kick-start the day. Research shows that people who eat breakfast have more energy all day long than people who don't eat breakfast. So come on, you. Up and at 'em.

No, really. I have no time. What can I do?

Grab a high-protein meal replacement powder (see Appendix A) and throw it in the blender. In 30 seconds it'll be blended and ready to go with you on the commuter train. And you can rip open a packet of instant oatmeal, put a little water in it, microwave it, put a spoon in it, and take that with you. If you've been planning your Lean Body meals—and I heartily urge that you do so—you already have food ready for the cooler.

Lee, you don't understand. I'm extremely late. In fact, while you were talking, I already hopped in the car. What do I do now?

Many drive-thru fast-food restaurants have Lean Body–friendly meals. (For a complete list, see page 98.) Or, hit a diner for egg whites and oatmeal, which will cover your protein and carbohydrate needs.

I forgot to mention something: I'm trapped in a two-hour market analysis meeting!

For situations like these, the best solution is to have a ready-to-drink protein shake handy (see Appendix A).

Today's going to be a really busy day. I just know I'm going to miss my workout. What can I do?

If you absolutely, positively have to miss a workout, pick up the next day where you left off. You've had a flat tire, but don't beat yourself up over it. Fix it and get back on the road tomorrow. It's a lifestyle we're trying to develop, so we need to be flexible.

But if this happens too often, you should really work on scheduling your workout into your day. First thing in the morning works best for a lot of people. Or be flexible about scheduling weight training or cardio if you can't make it to the gym. Go for a run or jump on your exercise bike, even if it was supposed to be a weight-training day.

(Sniff.) I've got a cold coming on. Should I work out?

The answer to that is no, in more cases than not. If you've got a sore throat and a general feeling of malaise, it's time to back off. Remember, we're making long-term life changes, not a quick-fix, lose-a-few-pounds bandage. Rest, pop some vitamins C and E, and stay away from sugar, because it depresses the immune system. We tend to catch colds when the immune system is compromised—too much sugar, alcohol, caffeine, not enough sleep. After a couple of days, do 20 minutes of light cardio and see how you feel. If you're okay, come back to the weight training the next day—but nothing too high intensity.

I'm sore. Should I work out?

A certain amount of soreness is normal and is to be expected, especially early in the program. But if you're really hurting, try warm, wet heat on the sore area for five to 10 minutes, switch to an ice bag for five to 10 minutes, then warm it back up again. Alternating the two creates a thermal pump: during vasodilation (the warmth), fresh blood flows in, then during vasoconstriction (the cold), blood is pushed out again. You're mechanically moving debris out of the area, which decreases your recuperation time. Just don't do this warm-cold-warm cycle more than two times; the thermal pump is something that should be used sparingly, like salt and exclamation points.

But should I still work out?

Yes. If you're tender to the touch, opt for some cardio to keep the blood moving—that's what's going to carry oxygen, remove debris, and heal your muscles—and try the thermal pump. Then pick up again the next day.

I've finished my workout, and now I feel like a million bucks. Should I do more?

No. (You were one of those overachievers in grade school always asking for extra credit, weren't you?) The key to this program is to use brief, intense exercise to stimulate the muscle. Any more can be counterproductive, putting you in a sorry state where you can't recover. You don't want to overtrain. Make a note on how you feel, then consider upping your training poundages the next time.

I've missed a meal, and I'm starving, but I have something bad in front of me. Something you warned me about back in the chapter on nutrition. Should I eat?

This answer may shock you: Eat a little. You may not be eating the most Lean Body–friendly foods, but you're better off snacking a little to tide your blood sugar over to the next meal. Select the food with the most protein—even if it's those little cocktail wieners—and have a half-size portion. Then wait 10 to 15 minutes so your stomach can feel satiated. Drink some water, which will help tide you over, too.

I'm up late watching a movie, and boy, do I have a craving.

It's important to realize that a craving isn't the same thing as actual hunger. Cravings are usually part of a pattern: You. TV. Favorite show. Oh yeah—bowl of ice cream. Sometimes, it's a programmed response that reaches back to childhood. What do you get when you've been a good little girl or boy? Cookies and milk, a candy bar, or some other kind of reward food.

Substitute the junk with something low in calories that will satisfy that innate craving. You might take the edge off by eating a cup of fat-free cottage cheese with low-calorie fruit, or some air-popped corn. (For more substitutions, see page 84).

I'm headed to a party tonight that'll be loaded with good friends, good music . . . and fatty and sugary food. What should I do? Sit home alone and play Tetris?

Plan ahead and eat a meal before the party. When you arrive, kiss your hosts on the cheeks and gravitate toward the low-fat snacks: the vegetable tray, the cocktail shrimp. Even a little rolled-up turkey with dry bread won't be too bad. Pop some olives, which have healthy fat. Whatever you do, stay away from chips, dips, fried snacks, alcohol, and the karaoke machine.

Lee, I'm in a funk. I just don't want to do the Lean Body thing today, okay?

If it's just one day, understand that all of us have off days. Maybe your boss chewed you out; maybe you got a parking ticket. Getting your blood flowing in the gym can be the best remedy, since it releases endorphins. Think of it as a workout upper—your seratonin levels go up and you are kicked out of your funk.

If you're still not feeling motivated, go ahead and pack it in and don't beat yourself up over it. If you're in a funk that lasts for days or even weeks, it may be that you're overtrained—you're doing more than your body can recover from. Lighten up or back off for a couple of days, then return to your regular routine. If you suspect that you may be clinically depressed, see your doctor. But if you're normally an upbeat person, it may be that you are overtrained or undernourished.

I'm traveling for business, I'm at the hotel, it's late . . . so what do I do now?

You can achieve a lean body even if you're 1,000 miles from home. Hopefully you prepared before you left—working out that morning, packing meals—but regardless, it's time for some recon work at the hotel. Look for a workout room at the hotel; an increasing number of hotels now have them. Enjoy a light snack. An apple and packets of instant oatmeal and protein powder can be used as emergency rations.

In the morning, go to the gym before you begin your day.

I'm on vacation. Should I keep going anyway?

The idea is to develop a lifestyle you can live with 24/7. If you're just starting out, and not yet in "maintaining" mode, try to avoid taking a vacation during those first 12 weeks. When you do take one, don't stress out about missing the routine for a week. Just make sure that your week off doesn't turn into two . . . then three. Resume the program the first day you're back.

My family isn't on the Lean Body nutrition program. Should I convert them?

You can't expect people to change their habits at the same time you change yours. So don't try to impose the nutrition program on others until they're willing. When they see you changing, they'll get interested. Don't lecture; just gently encourage them. In the meantime, satiate yourself on your own nutritious Lean Body food.

Today is my cheat meal day. I'm feeling great and want to skip it. Should I?

The answer is no. (Surprised?) It's tempting to want to give it 110 percent and say, *Forget the cheat meal! I can do without! Grrrrr!* But some 24, 36 hours later, you might not feel so superior, and you're more than likely to cave in to cravings. Eat some "normal" foods with your cheat meal, because that'll take care of any feelings of deprivation for the rest of the week. Just don't overdo it.

How about this: Can I bank two cheat meals and have them on the same day?

No. You're just setting yourself up to feel psychologically deprived later. And physically, you'd be overloading your system. The meal plan is about reprogramming yourself to make food no big deal. With small, frequent feedings, you have all of the amino acids and blood sugar you need. You won't get hungry.

What about skipping a meal to cut back on my total caloric intake?

Say it with me: No way. Allowing yourself to get hungry is the quickest way to fail. Admit it—everything starts looking good when you're in starvation mode. So eat like you should vote: early, and often.

It's week one, day six of the program. Why am I so cranky?

There are three possible reasons:

1. Your body's chemistry is changing—after all, you're fueling it differently these days—and you're going through a withdrawal process.

2. You might not be eating enough. Instead of eating fists and palms, add a "finger" to each and see if your mood improves.

3. You were already a cranky person before you started the Lean Body Promise.

I'm in week five of this program, I feel energetic, but I don't look any different. What's the deal?

Keep in mind that a lot of the changes in the first few weeks are taking place on the inside. There's a reason you feel more energetic: things are changing physiologically, and you're generating more energy through food and exercise. As for the visible rewards, have patience. A lot of times when you start losing body fat, the first five or 10 pounds comes off from around your internal organs first. It may be so gradual that you won't notice it. That's why I recommend the use of feedback, namely body fat calipers and update photos. (See Part Three, page 51, for more ways of tracking feedback.)

I'm a UPS guy who hauls boxes all day for a living. Do I really need to work out in my spare time?

A UPS guy might walk and haul boxes all day, but rarely does his heart rate reach over 150 beats per minute unless he's being chased by a dog. With bicycling and cardio workouts, your heart rate is kept up at a higher range for an extended period of time, which is a benefit to your heart and lungs. Plus, the workouts in the Lean Body program target particular body parts with brief, intense exercise and have a specific goal in mind. Random physical or manual labor may burn calories, but it won't do much for building optimal lean body mass.

I'm older. Can I still do this?

Of course. Consult with your doctor first and have a stress test—especially if you have high blood pressure, or are grossly overweight or extremely sedentary. But if you pass the test, this is a program you can grow into. And you can vary the intensity to suit your lifestyle.

I'm a young mother with kids. What about me?

This is the perfect opportunity to teach your kids about nutrition and fitness. (After all, Mom—along with Dad—you're one of their biggest role models.) Find a good gym with a childcare area where the kids will be entertained—or even led through some fitness classes—so you can squeeze a workout into your hectic schedule.

As far as food, it's never too early to start your children eating right. Kids should get used to eating small, frequent meals during the day. The only modification: Kids need a diet that's higher in carbs and essential fats than adults do. Simply put, they need more energy to run around and play dodgeball and chase the dog and do the million other things that healthy, active kids do.

It may be a battle at first, especially with older kids who are used to eating what they want whenever they want. But there are some strategies you can use. For instance, try chicken nuggets you bake in the oven, which have less fat than the fried kind. Substitute healthy snacks for overprocessed, sugary junk foods. Try fruit, fat-free cottage cheese, whole-grain crackers, and nuts. When it comes down to it, if that's all there is in the house, they'll get used to it.

I'm a vegetarian.

Excellent! The Lean Body program is compatible with a vegetarian diet. If you are a lacto-ovo vegetarian—you consume milk and egg products—you can use low-fat cottage cheese, protein drinks, and egg whites as your protein. If you're a vegan, you can still do the Lean Body plan by using soy protein. Just keep in mind that soy is an incomplete protein, which means it doesn't have all of the essential amino acids your body needs to produce other amino acids. That's easily remedied by adding other foods such as rice and beans to your soy diet.

A Powerful Lean Body Nutrition Success Tool for You

Eating five times per day may seem daunting at first. There's the issue of time, preparation, and even cost. I've developed a method that saves both time and money, while taking the guesswork out of eating right. It involves the use of a high-tech, nutritionally dense shake that my company, Labrada Nutrition, developed over a period of seven years. It's called, appropriately enough, the Lean Body Meal Replacement (MRP) shake, and it has helped thousands of people complete their Lean Body program. Almost all of the people who have finished my online Lean Body Challenge over the years are regular users of Lean Body MRP shakes.

There's a reason for that. Lean Body MRP shakes help you by making it quick and easy for you to consume the small, frequent meals required in the Lean Body Meal Plan. Most people who embark on my program aren't used to eating five or more times a day, and some don't have the time to prepare meals. Lean Body MRP shakes help you through the Lean Body program, especially at those times when you just can't consume a whole meal.

Better yet, the Lean Body MRP shake is a nutritional powerhouse. Imagine taking a sackful of groceries—vegetables, fruits, grains, and lean meats—and extracting all of the best nutrients out of them. Nutrients that your body needs in order to burn fat and build lean muscle. Now imagine having all of these good nutrients concentrated into a shake that tastes like soft-serve ice cream. You would have a scientifically engineered "functional superfood" that tastes great. That's what the Lean Body MRP shake is.

Lean Body MRP shakes are available in individual-size powder packets that you mix in a blender with ice water, or in convenient Ready-to-Drink (RTD) shakes that you just chill and drink.

I have personally used Lean Body shakes religiously every day for over seven years and they have played an important part in my ability to stay fit and lean over the long run. If you are busy, like I am, you will be glad to know that this is one powerful nutrition tool you can easily use every day to take the brainwork out of preparing meals, not to mention to help you stay disciplined and motivated.

It is possible for you to get great results on my program by just eating whole foods alone, especially if you have time to shop and prepare nutritious meals (I hope that you do at least part of the time!). But many of the thousands of people whom I have coached through my *Lean Body Coaching Club* (www.leanbodycoach.com) don't have time to fix and consume multiple meals throughout the day. For them, there are Lean Body shakes, a powerful success tool that makes the Lean Body lifestyle more practical. It may offer you similar benefits.

If you would like additional information about Lean Body shakes, call Labrada Nutrition at 1-800-832-9948 (Department LBP1), or log on to www.leanbodypromise.com or www.labrada.com.

APPENDIX B

The Daily Planners

The Lean Body Promise
Daily Workout Success Planner

Date: _____   Workout:_____

Body Part	Module[1]	Exercise	Set[2]	Weight	Reps	Rest[3]	Notes
• _____	1		1				
			2				
			3				
	2		1				
			2				
			3				
	3		1				
			2				
			3				
• _____	1		1				
			2				
			3				
	2		1				
			2				
			3				
• _____	1		1				
			2				
			3				
	2		1				
			2				
			3				

Workout A: Chest • Shoulders • Triceps

Workout B: Back • Biceps

Workout C: Legs • Abs

[1] Only the back workout (Workout B) will require three modules.

[2] On the third (last) set of each exercise, do as many reps as possible, to failure.

[3] Keep rest between sets to less than one minute, or as long as it takes to catch your breath.

The Lean Body Promise
Daily Workout Success Planner

Date: _January 2_   Workout: _A_

Body Part	Module[1]	Exercise	Set[2]	Weight	Reps	Rest[3]	Notes
Chest	1	Bench Press	1	150	10	1 Min	Felt strong today! Next time will increase weights.
			2	150	8	1 Min	
			3	150	6	1 Min	
	2	Incline Flys	1	35	10	u	
			2	35	8	u	
			3	35	6	u	
	3		1				
			2				
			3				
Shoulders	1	Standing Barbell Press	1	70	10	1 Min	70 lbs. on first set was too easy. Try Starting with 80 next time. Good Pump!
			2	80	8	1 Min	
			3	90	6	1 Min	
	2	Dumbbell Side Laterals	1	25	10	u	
			2	30	8	u	
			3	30	6	u	
Triceps	1	Lying Triceps Extension	1	60	10		Lightened up after 2nd set-got too heavy for 6 reps! Failed at 8 reps w/60 lbs.
			2	70	8		
			3	60	6		
	2	Triceps Pushdown	1	60	10		
			2	60	8		
			3	50	6		

Workout A: Chest • Shoulders • Triceps

Workout B: Back • Biceps

Workout C: Legs • Abs

[1] Only the back workout (Workout B) will require three modules.

[2] On the third (last) set of each exercise, do as many reps as possible, to failure.

[3] Keep rest between sets to less than one minute, or as long as it takes to catch your breath.

The Lean Body Promise
Nutrition Success Planner

Date: _____

Breakfast
Time:_____

P _____ Notes:

C _____

VSF _____

Mini-Meal
Time:_____

P _____ Notes:

C _____

VSF _____

Lunch
Time:_____

P _____ Notes:

C _____

VSF _____

Mini-Meal
Time:_____

P _____ Notes:

C _____

VSF _____

Dinner
Time:_____

P _____ Notes:

C _____

VSF _____

P=Protein Foods   C= Carbohydrate Foods   VSF= Vegetables, Salads, and Fruit

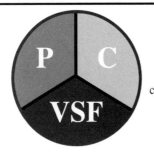

"Rule of Thirds"
Cover 1/3 of your plate with a protein, 1/3 with a
carb, and the final 1/3 with a vegetable, salad, or fruit.

The Lean Body Promise
Nutrition Success Planner

Date: _____

Breakfast
Time:_____

P _____   Notes:

C _____

VSF _____

Mini-Meal
Time:_____

P _____   Notes:

C _____

VSF _____

Lunch
Time:_____

P _____   Notes:

C _____

VSF _____

Mini-Meal
Time:_____

P _____   Notes:

C _____

VSF _____

Dinner
Time:_____

P _____   Notes:

C _____

VSF _____

P=Protein Foods   C= Carbohydrate Foods   VSF= Vegetables, Salads, and Fruit

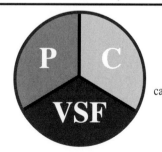

"Rule of Thirds"
Cover ⅓ of your plate with a protein, ⅓ with a carb, and the final ⅓ with a vegetable, salad, or fruit.

The Monthly Planners

The Lean Body Promise
Monthly Workout Success Planner

Month: _____

1	2	3	4	5	6	7
8	9	10	11	12	13	14
15	16	17	18	19	20	21
22	23	24	25	26	27	28
29	30	31				

A: Chest, Shoulders, Triceps

B: Back, Biceps

C: Legs, Abs

X: Cardio

O: Off

Notes: *Perform two consecutive days of weight training (A, B, or C), followed by one day of Cardio (X). Repeat this cycle, rotating the weight-training workouts (A, B, and C).

**If you take a day off (O), pick up with the next workout where you left off.

The Lean Body Promise
Monthly Workout Success Planner
Month: *January*

1	2	3	4	5	6	7
	A	*B*	*X*	*C*	*A*	*X*
8 B/X	**9** *C*	**10** *O*	**11** *A*	**12** *B*	**13** *X*	**14** *C*
15 *A*	**16** *X*	**17** B/X	**18** *C*	**19** *X*	**20** *A*	**21** *O*
22 *B*	**23** *X*	**24** *C*	**25** *A*	**26** *X*	**27** B/X	**28** *C*
29 *X*	**30** *O*	**31** *A*				

A: Chest, Shoulders, Triceps

B: Back, Biceps

C: Legs, Abs

X: Cardio

O: Off

Notes: *Perform two consecutive days of weight training (A, B, or C), followed by one day of Cardio (X). Repeat this cycle, rotating the weight-training workouts (A, B, and C).

**If you take a day off (O), pick up with the next workout where you left off.

Using Your Fat Calipers

Ever try to measure your own body fat by taking your love handles and "pinching an inch"? If you combine that popular method with a simple set of fat calipers, you'll actually have one of the most scientific ways of measuring body fat—and, more important, of tracking your lean body as it emerges.

The principle is called *skin-fold measurement*, and it's based on the fact that the majority of your body fat rests under your skin. Measure fat in one key area, and it'll give you a clear idea of how much body fat you have overall. To take your skin-fold measurement, you'll need a pair of inexpensive Accu-Measure skin-fold calipers. You can take your body fat measurement in three easy steps:

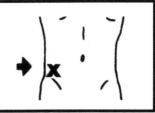
Figure #1

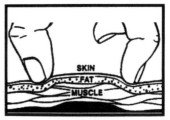
Figure #2

1. *Find the suprailiac site, located about one inch above your right hip bone.*

2. *Pull the skin and underlying fat away from the muscle tissue. While standing, firmly squeeze this skin*

fold between your left thumb and forefinger. Now place the jaws of the fat calipers over the skin fold.

3. *Press on the calipers until you hear a click. Release the jaws of the calipers and read your measurement in millimeters. Find your corresponding body fat percentage in the chart on page 209.*

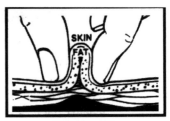

Figure #3

This is the number you'll use (along with your body weight) to track your progress. Plug these numbers into the handy Success Tracking Chart that follows, and you'll have a clear vision of how much fat you're blasting away, week by week.

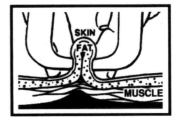

Figure #4

You can get your own Accu-Measure body fat calipers by calling call Labrada Nutrition at 1-800-832-9948 (Department LBP1), or log on to www.lean bodypromise.com or www.labrada.com.

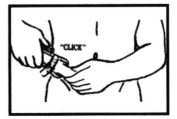

Figure #5

BODY FAT % MEASUREMENT CHART FOR MEN

Accu-Measure® Reading in Millimeters

	2-3	4-5	6-7	8-9	10-11	12-13	14-15	16-17	18-19	20-21	22-23	24-25	26-27	28-29	30-31	32-33	34-36
Up to 20	2.0	3.9	6.2	8.5	10.5	12.5	14.3	16.0	17.5	18.9	20.2	21.3	22.3	23.1	23.8	24.3	24.9
21-25	2.5	4.9	7.3	9.5	11.6	13.6	15.4	17.0	18.6	20.0	21.2	22.3	23.3	24.2	24.9	25.4	25.8
26-30	3.5	6.0	8.4	10.6	12.7	14.6	16.4	18.1	19.6	21.0	22.3	23.4	24.4	25.2	25.9	26.5	26.9
31-35	4.5	7.1	9.4	11.7	13.7	15.7	17.5	19.2	20.7	22.1	23.4	24.5	25.5	26.3	27.0	27.5	28.0
36-40	5.6	8.1	10.5	12.7	14.8	16.8	18.6	20.2	21.8	23.2	24.4	25.6	26.5	27.4	28.1	28.6	29.0
41-45	6.7	9.2	11.5	13.8	15.9	17.8	19.6	21.3	22.8	24.7	25.5	26.6	27.6	28.4	29.1	29.7	30.1
46-50	7.7	10.2	12.6	14.8	16.9	18.9	20.7	22.4	23.9	25.3	26.6	27.7	28.7	29.5	30.2	30.7	31.2
51-55	8.8	11.3	13.7	15.9	18.0	20.0	21.8	23.4	25.0	26.4	27.6	28.7	29.7	30.6	31.2	31.8	32.2
56 & UP	9.9	12.4	14.7	17.0	19.1	21.0	22.8	24.5	26.0	27.4	28.7	29.8	30.8	31.6	32.3	32.9	33.3
	LEAN				IDEAL				AVERAGE				ABOVE AVERAGE				

1) Obtain your % body fat measurement in millimeters using the Accu-Measure Body Fat Tester.
2) Find where the column with your body fat range intersects with the row with your age range.
3) The number at this intersection is your body fat percentage.

BODY FAT % MEASUREMENT CHART FOR WOMEN

Accu-Measure® Reading in Millimeters

	2-3	4-5	6-7	8-9	10-11	12-13	14-15	16-17	18-19	20-21	22-23	24-25	26-27	28-29	30-31	32-33	34-36
Up to 20	11.3	13.5	15.7	17.7	19.7	21.5	23.2	24.8	26.3	27.7	29.0	30.2	31.3	32.3	33.1	33.9	34.6
21-25	11.9	14.2	16.3	18.4	20.3	22.1	23.8	25.5	27.0	28.4	29.6	30.8	31.9	32.9	33.8	34.5	35.2
26-30	12.5	14.8	16.9	19.0	20.9	22.7	24.5	26.1	27.6	29.0	30.3	31.5	32.5	33.5	34.4	35.2	35.8
31-35	13.2	15.4	17.6	19.6	21.5	23.4	25.1	26.7	28.2	29.6	30.9	32.1	33.2	34.1	35.0	35.8	36.4
36-40	13.8	16.0	18.2	20.2	22.2	24.0	25.7	27.3	28.8	30.2	31.5	32.7	33.8	34.8	35.6	36.4	37.0
41-45	14.4	16.7	18.8	20.8	22.8	24.6	26.3	27.9	29.4	30.8	32.1	33.3	34.4	35.4	36.3	37.0	37.7
46-50	15.0	17.3	19.4	21.5	23.4	25.2	26.9	28.6	30.1	31.5	32.8	34.0	35.0	36.0	36.9	37.6	38.3
51-55	15.6	17.9	20.0	22.1	24.0	25.9	27.6	29.2	30.7	32.1	33.4	34.6	35.6	36.6	37.5	38.3	38.9
56 & UP	16.3	18.5	20.7	22.7	24.6	26.5	28.2	29.8	31.3	32.7	34.0	35.2	36.3	37.2	38.1	38.9	39.5
	LEAN				IDEAL				AVERAGE				ABOVE AVERAGE				

1) Obtain your % body fat measurement in millimeters using the Accu-Measure Body Fat Tester.
2) Find where the column with your body fat range intersects with the row with your age range.
3) The number at this intersection is your body fat percentage.

Using Your Fat Calipers   209

The Lean Body Promise
Success Tracking Chart

Week	Body Weight[1] (lbs)	%Body Fat[2]	Body Fat[3] (lbs)	Lean Weight[4] (lbs)
1				
2				
3				
4				
5				
6				
7				
8				
9				
10				
11				
12				

Example: [1] Body Weight = 200 lbs.

[2] BF% = 25% (.25)

[3] Pounds Body Fat = Body Weight × BF%
= (200) × (.25)
= 50 Pounds Fat

[4] Pounds Lean Weight = Body Weight—Pounds Body Fat
= 200—50
= 150 Pounds Lean

Seven Days
of Lean Body Meals

Confused by all of the healthy choices you have in front of you? Let me take the guess-work out of your first week. Here's a complete sample menu for your first seven days on the Lean Body Meal Plan. (You'll find recipes for many of these delicious dishes starting on page 215.) If you don't feel like cooking anything fancy, remember that pre-cooked chicken breasts, baked yams, whole-grain rice, vegetables, and fruits are just some of the foods you can use to throw together a Lean Body meal when pressed for time.

DAY ONE

BREAKFAST: Scrambled egg whites, Homemade Muesli (page 230), coffee

MIDMORNING SNACK: Lean Body Ready-to-Drink (RTD) Shake (vanilla), Yam Muffin (page 221)

LUNCH: Chicken breast sandwich, apple, small handful of pecans, iced tea

MIDAFTERNOON: Lean Body RTD Shake (chocolate), banana

DINNER: Grilled halibut, small baked potato, salad with olive oil and balsamic vinegar, frozen yogurt, water

DAY TWO

BREAKFAST: Creamy Salmon Omelet (page 227), two slices of whole-grain toast, coffee

MIDMORNING SNACK: Lean Body Protein Bar, apple, water

LUNCH: Chicken and Veggie Burrito (page 215), small salad with olive oil, honeydew melon slice, iced tea

MIDAFTERNOON: Lean Body RTD Shake (chocolate)

DINNER: Polenta and Sea Scallops (page 216), Grilled Veggies (page 222), raspberry sorbet, water

DAY THREE

BREAKFAST: Breakfast Burrito (page 228), banana, coffee

MIDMORNING SNACK: One cup of fat-free cottage cheese, sliced strawberries, granola bar

LUNCH: Tuna sandwich, small salad with olive oil, apple slices, diet soda

MIDAFTERNOON: Lean Body RTD Shake (vanilla), Yam Muffin, nuts

DINNER: Turkey Tenderloins and Rosemary Potatoes (page 223), Grilled Veggies, small salad with nonfat dressing, water

DAY FOUR

BREAKFAST: Lean Body MRP Shake (mix vanilla in the blender with strawberries and a banana)

MIDMORNING SNACK: Lean Body RTD Shake (chocolate)

LUNCH: Turkey Tenderloins (from the night before), Lentil Soup (page 220), Tangy New Potatoes (page 229), iced tea

MIDAFTERNOON: One cup of fat-free cottage cheese, peach slices, granola bar, water

DINNER: Sweet Potato Salmon (page 226), Tangy New Potatoes, small salad, frozen yogurt, water

DAY FIVE

BREAKFAST: Scrambled egg whites with low-fat Cheddar cheese, one cup of oatmeal, half cup of blueberries, coffee

MIDMORNING SNACK: Lean Body Protein Bar, apple, water

LUNCH: Sweet Potato Salmon (from the night before), Lentil Soup, iced tea

MIDAFTERNOON: Lean Body RTD Shake (chocolate), Yam Muffin, nuts

DINNER: Cajun Tuna with Black Beans (page 219), Wild Rice with Cranberries and Pecans (page 229), small salad, one cup of mixed berries, water

DAY SIX

BREAKFAST: Lean Body MRP Shake (mix vanilla in the blender with one teaspoon of instant coffee), small bowl of Total flakes with skim milk

MIDMORNING SNACK: One cup of fat-free cottage cheese, Yam Muffin, water

LUNCH: Mediterranean Sandwich (page 224), small salad with olive oil, one cup of Wild Rice with Cranberries and Pecans (from the night before), iced tea

MIDAFTERNOON: Lean Body RTD Shake (vanilla), banana, nuts

DINNER: Sweet Mustard Chicken with Creole Vegetables (page 225), baked sweet potato, small salad with olive oil, raspberry sorbet, water

Day Seven

BREAKFAST: Breakfast Burrito, honeydew melon, coffee

MIDMORNING SNACK: Lean Body RTD Shake (chocolate), Yam Muffin

LUNCH: Sweet Mustard Chicken with Creole Vegetables (from the night before), baked sweet potato, small salad with olive oil, iced tea

MIDAFTERNOON: One cup of fat-free cottage cheese, sliced peaches, nuts, water

DINNER: Grilled red snapper, Tangy New Potatoes, small salad, one cup of mixed berries, water

Lean Body–Friendly Recipes

Chicken and Veggie Burritos

ESTIMATED PREP TIME: 5 MINUTES   ESTIMATED COOK TIME: 10 MINUTES

1 cooked boneless, skinless chicken breast (roasted or grilled, marinated)

1 cup cooked brown rice

½ large portabella mushroom cap, wiped clean

¼ large red onion

½ large roasted red bell pepper

1 tablespoon olive oil

½ teaspoon minced fresh garlic

4 corn or low-carb tortillas

Medium skillet; microwave

1. Grab your chicken and rice from the fridge.

2. Cut the mushroom, onion, and pepper into thin slices. Heat the oil in a medium skillet, and add the mushroom, onion, pepper, and garlic. Sauté until the onion is soft, about 5 minutes.

3. Slice the chicken, add it to the skillet with the rice, and gently stir to combine everything. Cook just long enough for all to get hot.

4. Warm the tortillas in the microwave and heap the mixture on them. Roll up burrito-style.

Try adding fresh cilantro or salsa.

makes 4 servings

Polenta and Sea Scallops

ESTIMATED PREP TIME: **5** MINUTES

ESTIMATED COOK TIME: **15** MINUTES

---

1 chicken bouillon cube

2 cups quick-cooking polenta (corn grits, found in health food store or pasta section)

½ large red onion

1 large portabella mushroom cap, wiped clean

½ large roasted red bell pepper

2 tablespoons olive oil, plus extra as needed

1 pound sea scallops

¼ cup freshly grated Parmesan cheese

1 teaspoon of minced fresh garlic

Medium saucepan; medium skillet; large nonstick skillet

---

1. Bring 6 cups of water to a boil in a medium saucepan. Stir in the bouillon cube and polenta. Turn the heat down and simmer, stirring occasionally, until creamy, about 10 minutes.

2. Meanwhile, cut the onion, mushroom, and pepper into thin slices. Heat the oil in a medium skillet and add them to the skillet along with the garlic. Sauté until the onions are soft, 4 to 5 minutes. Set aside.

3. Dry the scallops well on paper towels. Place a little olive oil in a large nonstick skillet and heat it until very hot; add the scallops in a single layer. This needs to be done on high heat so they cook quickly and seal on the outside. Cook the scallops about 2 minutes on each side. Do not overcook; the scallops should cut easily with a fork. Remove from the heat immediately.

4. In large bowls layer the polenta, cheese, and veggies, and top with the scallops.

〉〉   makes 4 servings

Chicken in a Bag

ESTIMATED PREP TIME: **10** MINUTES   ESTIMATED COOK TIME: **60** MINUTES

This is a dish you can prep ahead of time and place in the fridge. Pop it in the oven when you get home. You can also increase the ingredients to make as many servings as you want for lunches or another dinner.

1 pound boneless, skinless chicken breasts
¼ cup whole-wheat flour
3 large red potatoes, washed and cut into chunks
1 small white onion, coarsely chopped
1 pound baby carrots
8 mushrooms, wiped clean and sliced thick
2 chicken bouillon cubes
1 teaspoon minced fresh garlic
2 bay leaves
1 teaspoon dried thyme
Dash of pepper
1 cup white wine
Large cooking bag; 9- by 13-inch baking pan

1. Preheat the oven to 350 degrees.

2. Rinse the chicken breasts with cold water and pat dry with paper towels. Sprinkle both sides with the flour.

3. Set the cooking bag in the baking pan. Into the bag, place the chicken, potatoes, onion, carrots, and mushrooms.

4. In a microwave-safe cup, heat the bouillon cubes with 1 cup of water on high for 1 minute. Stir to dissolve the cubes, and add the garlic, bay leaves, thyme, and pepper. Pour this over the chicken and vegetables, along with the wine. Close the bag with its tie. (If you're prepping this in the morning, put the bag in the fridge still sitting in the baking dish.)

5. Place in the oven and bake for 60 minutes.

» makes 4 servings

Quick "Lasagna"

ESTIMATED PREP TIME: **5** MINUTES   ESTIMATED COOK TIME: **15** MINUTES

---

1 package bow tie pasta (1 pound)

1 tablespoon olive oil

¼ cup chopped onion

1 teaspoon minced fresh garlic

1 pound extra lean ground beef or ground turkey breast

Salt and pepper

1 cup low-fat cottage cheese

2 tablespoons shredded Parmesan cheese

Large pasta pot; large skillet

---

1. Bring a large pot of water to a boil. Add the pasta and cook according to the package directions. When done, drain well.

2. Meanwhile, heat the oil in a large skillet. Add the onion and garlic and sauté until the onion is soft, about 5 minutes.

3. Add the beef and cook, stirring to break up clumps, until the meat is cooked through, about 10 minutes. (There should be no grease to drain.) Add salt and pepper to taste.

4. Add the cottage cheese and mix well. It will start getting gooey.

5. Divide the pasta into bowls. Spoon the meat mixture on top, and sprinkle with the Parmesan cheese.

Cajun Tuna with Black Beans

ESTIMATED PREP TIME: 10 MINUTES

ESTIMATED COOK TIME: 5 MINUTES

Look for dark red/purple tuna. You can also cook the tuna on the grill over high heat.

---

1 cup cooked sushi rice

1 can (about 15 ounces) ranch-style black beans

2 fresh ahi tuna steaks, 4 to 6 ounces each

Cajun seasoning

Olive oil

1 Roma or plum tomato, chopped

¼ small white onion, chopped

Fresh cilantro

Small saucepan; small skillet

---

1. Pull the rice out of the fridge and divide onto 2 plates. Set aside.

2. Pour the beans into a saucepan and warm.

3. Sprinkle each side of the tuna with the Cajun seasoning. Drizzle a small amount of oil into the skillet and heat the oil until very hot. Add the tuna and sear it about 2 minutes on each side. Do not overcook! The tuna should still be pink on the inside.

4. While the tuna is cooking, heat the rice in the microwave.

5. As soon as the tuna is cooked, remove it from the heat. Place a serving of beans on top of the rice, top with a piece of tuna, and garnish with the tomato, onion, and cilantro.

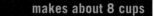
Lentil Soup

ESTIMATED PREP TIME: 10 MINUTES

ESTIMATED COOK TIME: 60 MINUTES

This makes enough for several meals. And it's great reheated.

---

6 ounces ground turkey breast

3 beef bouillon cubes

5 Roma or plum tomatoes, coarsely chopped

8 to 10 mushrooms, cut in halves or quarters depending on size

2 bay leaves

1 teaspoon minced fresh garlic

4 "shakes" pepper

1½ cup dried lentils

Large soup or pasta pot

---

1. In a large pot, cook the turkey over low heat just until it stops looking raw. Stir while it's cooking to break up clumps.

2. Add 6 cups of water and bring to a boil. Add the bouillon cubes, tomatoes, mushrooms, bay leaves, garlic, pepper, and lentils. Bring back to a boil, then turn down to a low simmer. Cook about 1 hour, stirring occasionally to prevent sticking on the bottom. The soup will thicken as the lentils soften and dissolve.

Serve with fresh whole-grain bread.

Yam Muffins

ESTIMATED PREP TIME: 10 MINUTES

ESTIMATED COOK TIME: 30 TO 35 MINUTES

Feel free to mix in dried cherries, nuts, chopped figs, peaches, or dates.

2½ cups oat bran

1 teaspoon baking soda

1 teaspoon double-acting baking powder

1 teaspoon ground allspice

1 teaspoon ground cinnamon

1 large yam (sweet potato), peeled and shredded

8 egg whites

1 cup molasses

1½ cups unsweetened applesauce

¼ cup vegetable oil

Large mixing bowl; small mixing bowl; muffin tin with 18 cups; foil muffin liners (optional)

---

1. Preheat the oven to 350 degrees.

2. In a large mixing bowl, stir together the oat bran, baking soda, baking powder, allspice, and cinnamon. In a small bowl, mix the shredded yam, egg whites, molasses, applesauce, and oil. Pour the wet mixture into the dry mixture, and stir to mix thoroughly.

3. Fill muffin cups about level (I use the foil liners for no mess or sticking). Bake for 30 to 35 minutes. Test with a toothpick; it should come out with nothing sticking to it. If the muffins need more time, put them back for a few minutes, then test again.

Grilled Veggies

ESTIMATED PREP TIME: 15 MINUTES

ESTIMATED COOK TIME: 10 MINUTES

Use extras for quick garnishes on main dishes.

---

1 eggplant
1 green zucchini
1 yellow zucchini or yellow squash
1 red bell pepper
1 green bell pepper
10 large mushrooms
1 red onion, peeled
1 bunch asparagus
¼ cup olive oil
1 tablespoon minced fresh garlic
½ teaspoon sea salt
4 "shakes" pepper
Small mixing bowl; 2 gallon-size plastic bags; veggie grill basket

---

1. Turn the grill on high.

2. Wash all veggies. Slice the eggplant into ½-inch circles, then cut into halves. Cut off the ends of the squashes and slice into ½-inch circles. Cut the mushrooms in half. Remove the stems and bottoms of the peppers; slice them open; discard the seeds and cut the flesh into large squares. Cut the onions into ½-inch wedges, but do not pull the layers apart. Break off the heavy stems of the asparagus, then cut the asparagus in half.

3. Combine the oil, garlic, salt, and pepper, and divide between the two bags. Put half of each vegetable into each bag. Zip closed and shake to coat the veggies with the oil mixture.

4. Place the veggie grill basket on the grill and put in the vegetables. Toss to cook evenly for about 10 minutes. The veggies are best if a little charred but still crunchy.

Serve hot sprinkled with grated Parmesan cheese, or cold drizzled with balsamic vinegar.

Turkey Tenderloins and Rosemary Potatoes

ESTIMATED PREP TIME: 5 MINUTES (NOT INCLUDING MARINATING TIME)
ESTIMATED COOK TIME: 20 MINUTES

The turkey is best if you marinate it overnight. You can cut the potatoes into chunks or thin slices, or however you prefer; the smaller you cut the potatoes, the faster they will cook.

---

1 chicken bouillon cube, dissolved in ¼ cup water
3 turkey breast tenderloins (solid turkey breast), about 1 pound total
1 cup milk
1 teaspoon minced fresh garlic
Salt and pepper
4 tablespoons olive oil
4 red new potatoes, washed
½ teaspoon crumbled dried rosemary
Garlic salt
Gallon-size plastic freezer bag set in a large bowl; 2 large skillets

---

1. Dissolve the bouillon cube in ¼ cup boiling water; set aside to cool.
2. Slice the turkey crosswise into ½-inch medallions. Place the turkey in the plastic bag with the bouillon, milk, garlic, and salt and pepper. Zip shut and refrigerate. Marinate for at least 8 hours, up to a full day.

3. Drain the turkey and discard the marinade. Pour 2 tablespoons olive oil into a large skillet over medium-high heat; when hot, add the turkey. Cook until the turkey is no longer pink; you want to sear but not burn it.

4. Meanwhile in another large skillet, heat 2 tablespoons olive oil. Add the potatoes, rosemary, and garlic salt to taste. Sauté on medium-high heat, stirring frequently until soft.

Mediterranean Sandwiches

ESTIMATED PREP TIME: **10** MINUTES   ESTIMATED COOK TIME: **10** MINUTES

The chicken can be freshly grilled, or use roasted chicken you have in the fridge.

Whole-grain focaccia bread or 4 slices any other crusty whole-grain bread
Olive oil
1 roasted red pepper from the jar, drained well and sliced
1 portabella mushroom cap, wiped clean and sliced
6 black Greek olives, pitted and chopped
¼ small red onion, sliced
1 large cooked boneless, skinless chicken breast, sliced on the diagonal
1 tablespoon soft goat cheese
Large skillet

---

1. Slice the focaccia to make 2 sandwiches. Brush with a little olive oil on the cut side and set aside.

2. In a large skillet, drizzle a little olive oil. Heat over medium-high heat, then add the pepper, mushroom, olives, and onion. Cook, stirring frequently, until the onion is crisp-tender. Add the chicken and toss together. Remove from the skillet and set aside.

3. Place the bread in the skillet, oiled-side down, and grill for 2 to 3 minutes. Remove and spread the goat cheese on each slice. Top with the chicken and vegetable mixture.

Sweet Mustard Chicken with Creole Vegetables

ESTIMATED PREP TIME: 10 MINUTES (NOT INCLUDING MARINATING TIME)

ESTIMATED COOK TIME: 30 MINUTES

The chicken is best if marinated for a few hours. When grilling the chicken, be careful that the coating does not burn before the chicken is cooked through.

3 tablespoons Dijon mustard

3 tablespoons brown sugar

½ teaspoon ground ginger

½ cup white wine

4 boneless, skinless chicken breasts

Olive oil

4 cups fresh green beans (about 40), washed and ends cut off

½ red onion

2 Roma or plum tomatoes, chopped

White pepper

Garlic salt

Gallon-size plastic freezer bag; large skillet

1. Combine the mustard, sugar, ginger, and wine in the plastic bag. Squish until mixed thoroughly, add the chicken, and squish to coat well. Set aside for at least 30 minutes to marinate, or refrigerate for up to a full day.

2. When you're ready to cook, preheat the grill. Place the chicken on the grill and cook, turning once, until no longer pink inside. Do not overcook! If the coating starts to burn, move the chicken to the side, away from the heat.

3. While the chicken is grilling, heat the olive oil in a large skillet. Add the beans and the onion. Cook until the beans are almost soft, about 30 minutes. Add the tomatoes, and sprinkle with pepper and garlic salt to taste. Continue cooking until the tomatoes are dissolving.

Sweet Potato Salmon

ESTIMATED PREP TIME: 10 MINUTES

ESTIMATED COOK TIME: 25 MINUTES

---

2 yams (sweet potatoes)

2 tablespoons brown sugar

½ teaspoon ground cinnamon

2 large salmon fillets, skin on, about 8 ounces each

1 teaspoon butter

1 bag (10 ounces) fresh spinach, rinsed and drained

1 tablespoon olive oil

6 pecan halves, chopped

Medium saucepan; handheld mixer; grill or heavy medium skillet; large skillet with
a cover

---

1. Peel the yams and cut them into large chunks. Place them in a saucepan, cover with water, bring to a boil, and cook until soft, 15 to 20 minutes. Remove from the heat, drain, add the sugar and cinnamon, and whip with a handheld mixer until fluffy. Set aside and keep warm.

2. While the yams are cooking, heat the grill or a heavy skillet. Rinse the salmon and pat it dry with paper towels. Place it skin-side down on the grill and top each piece with half of the butter. Cook undisturbed until the salmon flakes easily, about 10 to 15 minutes; do not turn.

3. Just before the salmon is done, heat the oil in a large skillet over high heat. Add the spinach, cover, and cook, shaking the pan occasionally, about 2 minutes. (You want the spinach to wilt and shrink, but not become soggy.)

4. Place a scoop of mashed yams on each serving plate. Top with spinach. Slide a spatula between the fish and the skin, and lift off the fish. Place the fish on the spinach. (You can remove the skin from the grill and discard it after dinner.) Sprinkle with the chopped pecans and serve.

Creamy Salmon Omelet

ESTIMATED PREP TIME: 5 MINUTES ESTIMATED COOK TIME: 10 MINUTES

You can find packaged smoked salmon in the deli or fish department.

1 tablespoon olive oil
¼ small red onion, chopped fine
1 small handful fresh spinach leaves, washed and dried
1 tablespoon fat-free cream cheese
2 ounces smoked salmon, chopped coarsely
Chopped fresh dill
5 jumbo egg whites
Small nonstick skillet; small bowl

1. Heat the olive oil in the skillet, and add the onion. Sauté a few minutes; add the spinach, and stir until the spinach is wilted. Add the cream cheese, salmon, and a sprinkle of dill; stir until combined. Set aside in a small bowl.

2. Do not clean the skillet. Pour in the egg whites and cook in flat omelet form over low heat, lifting the edges for the liquid part to run underneath. When cooked, place the salmon mixture on top and fold over.

Serve with whole-grain toast.

Breakfast Burritos

ESTIMATED PREP TIME: 5 MINUTES   ESTIMATED COOK TIME: 10 MINUTES

Olive oil
1 medium potato, cooked in the microwave and chopped into small pieces
¼ onion, chopped fine
Garlic salt
Pepper
8 egg whites
4 corn or low-carb tortillas
Medium nonstick skillet

1. Heat the olive oil in the skillet over medium heat and add the potato and onion. Cook, stirring occasionally, until the onion is soft, about 5 minutes. Sprinkle with garlic salt and pepper to taste.
2. Add the egg whites and cook, scrambling, until done to taste.
3. Warm the tortillas in the microwave. Spoon the mixture on top and roll up. Serve while still warm, or wrap in foil to take with you.

Serve plain or with salsa and/or low-fat cheese.

Tangy New Potatoes

ESTIMATED PREP TIME: 5 MINUTES (NOT INCLUDING COOLING TIME)

ESTIMATED COOK TIME: 15 MINUTES

---

8 to 10 small red new potatoes
2 tablespoons Dijon mustard
1 tablespoon balsamic vinegar
1 tablespoon olive oil
½ teaspoon white pepper
½ small red onion, chopped fine
Medium saucepan; large bowl

---

1. Wash the potatoes thoroughly and cut into small cubes. Place in the saucepan, cover with water, and bring to a boil. Cook until just tender, 10 to 15 minutes. (Do not overcook; keep firm.) Drain, rinse, drain again, and let cool.

2. Mix the mustard, vinegar, oil, pepper, and onion in a large bowl. Add the potatoes and toss gently to coat. Cover and refrigerate. Serve cold.

Wild Rice with Cranberries and Pecans

ESTIMATED PREP TIME: 5 MINUTES   ESTIMATED COOK TIME: 45 MINUTES

Serve hot as a side dish, or let this cool before you portion it into plastic bags for future meals.

---

2 cups short-grain brown rice
½ cup wild rice

2 bouillon cubes
1 cup dried cranberries
1 cup coarsely chopped pecans
Fine-mesh strainer; medium saucepan with cover

1. Place the brown rice and wild rice in a strainer and rinse under cold water. Drain thoroughly.

2. Combine the rices and bouillon cubes in the saucepan with 5 cups of water. Bring to a boil. Stir once, cover, and turn heat down to low. Cook the rice at a slow bubble until all the water has been absorbed.

3. Stir in the cranberries and pecans.

›› makes about 7½ cups

Homemade Muesli

ESTIMATED PREP TIME: 5 MINUTES

This beats the oats out of the boxed variety!

4 cups whole oats
1 cup crisped rice cereal
½ cup coarsely chopped pecans
½ cup coarsely chopped raw almonds (skin on)
½ cup raw sunflower seeds
½ cup dried cherries
½ cup golden raisins
Large mixing bowl; large storage container with close-fitting cover

Mix all ingredients in a large bowl. Store tightly covered.

Scoop a serving into a bowl and add skim milk (and sugar substitute, if you like).

Your Lean Body Fridge List

The Plan: Eat five meals made up of the following components every day—basically, a meal every three hours. Think of it as breakfast, lunch, and dinner, with a snack or mini-meal at midmorning and midafternoon.

The Lean Body Promise
Fridge Reminder List

Protein

How much?
A portion the size of your open hand.

- ☐ egg whites or egg substitutes
- ☐ chicken breast
- ☐ turkey breast
- ☐ lean ground turkey breast
- ☐ cod
- ☐ crab
- ☐ flounder
- ☐ haddock
- ☐ halibut
- ☐ red snapper
- ☐ salmon*
- ☐ scallops
- ☐ shrimp
- ☐ sole
- ☐ tuna*
- ☐ fat-free cottage cheese
- ☐ protein powder
  (CarbWatchers ProPlete, ProV60)
- ☐ Lean Body Meal Replacement Powder
  Packets Ready-to-Drink Shakes and Bars)

Vegetables

How much?
As much as you want,
but at least one-third
of your plate.

- ☐ lettuce and leafy greens
- ☐ broccoli
- ☐ cauliflower
- ☐ green beans
- ☐ carrots
- ☐ spinach
- ☐ asparagus
- ☐ artichokes
- ☐ peppers
- ☐ tomatoes
- ☐ peas
- ☐ cabbage
- ☐ zucchini
- ☐ cucumbers
- ☐ squash
- ☐ onions
- ☐ mushrooms

Carbs

How much?
A portion the size of
your closed fist.

- ☐ oatmeal
- ☐ whole-grain cooked cereal
- ☐ Cream of Wheat
- ☐ brown rice
- ☐ wild rice
- ☐ new potatoes (with skin)
- ☐ sweet potatoes
- ☐ yams
- ☐ beans
- ☐ corn
- ☐ peas
- ☐ rice cakes
- ☐ lentils
- ☐ black-eyed peas
- ☐ whole-grain pasta and bread**
- ☐ corn tortillas

Lean Body Desserts

How much?
No more than two to three servings
per day.

- ☐ cherries
- ☐ grapefruit
- ☐ berries (blue, black, rasp, straw)
- ☐ peaches
- ☐ apricots
- ☐ oranges
- ☐ pears
- ☐ plums
- ☐ tangerines
- ☐ apples
- ☐ grapes***
- ☐ raisins***
- ☐ mangoes***
- ☐ melons (cantaloupe, honeydew)***
- ☐ dates***
- ☐ figs***
- ☐ pineapple ***
- ☐ bananas***

Lean Body Good Fats

How much?
Add two servings per day.

- ☐ flaxseed oil
- ☐ salmon, mackerel, sardines
- ☐ fish oils
- ☐ walnuts, almonds, cashews,
  other nuts and seeds

- ☐ avocadoes
- ☐ olive oil
- ☐ olives

Notes:
* may contain higher levels of fat
**You should limit these carbs
***higher in sugar, and hence should be eaten sparingly

Index

About the Author

One of the world's best known and most celebrated bodybuilding legends, Lee Labrada brings real-life experience to the nutrition and exercise techniques presented in *The Lean Body Promise*. Lee's approach is meant to appeal to anyone interested in making positive physical changes, not just to the elite athlete.

Lee holds twenty-two professional bodybuilding titles, including Mr. Universe. He is one of only four men in history to consistently place in the top four at the Mr. Olympia competition (the "Super Bowl" of bodybuilding) for seven consecutive years—a feat he shares with Arnold Schwarzenegger. In 2004, Lee was inducted into the IFBB Pro Bodybuilding Hall of Fame. He has appeared on the covers of more than 100 magazines worldwide and has appeared as a fitness and nutrition expert on ABC's *Extreme Makeover,* CNBC, FOX, NBC, CBS, CNN, WGN, and ESPN.

Lee credits his success to work ethic and dedication that he learned from his parents. The family escaped the Communist regime in Cuba when Lee was just two years old. Lee learned early on that anything is possible in America if you are willing to work hard and work smart. Lee's desire to help others reach their health and nutrition goals inspired him to found Labrada Nutrition, and to create a line of award-winning nutrition and supplement products. Equally successful in business as he is in the gym, Lee turned his Labrada Nutrition into one of the fastest-growing privately held companies in the United States—earning Inc. 500 status after only six years. Over the past few years, more than 60,000 people have taken advantage of Lee's exceptional nutrition education by subscribing to his free online newsletter at www.leanbodycoach.com.

In June 2002, Lee was appointed the first fitness czar in the city of Houston, where he helped launch Get Lean Houston!, a health and fitness campaign designed to get the city's residents into better shape. Lee is credited with helping Houston shed the dubious title of "America's Fattest City."

Lee holds a bachelor's degree in civil engineering from the University of Houston and lives in Houston, Texas, with his wife and three young sons. Lee Labrada is available for corporate fitness seminars and speaking engagements. For more information, contact Lee at lee@labrada.com.

Lee's Bodybuilding Titles

I don't include this list to toot my own horn. Just consider this list as part of the résumé I'm handing you while applying for the job of being your personal fitness trainer. I'm proud of my credentials, but more importantly, I hope they inspire you to put your faith in me.

1982 NPC Texas Collegiate Championships (1st Place)
1982 NPC Junior Gulf Coast Championships (1st Place)
1983 NPC Texas Championships, 1st Middleweight and Overall
1984 NPC USA Bodybuilding Championships (2nd Place, Light Heavyweight)
1984 NPC National Bodybuilding Championships (5th Place, Middleweight)
1985 NPC National Bodybuilding Championships (1st Place, Middleweight)
1985 IFBB Mr. Universe (1st Place)

1986	IFBB Night of Champions (1st Place)
1987	IFBB Pro World Cup (2nd Place)
1987	IFBB Mr. Olympia (3rd Place)
1987	IFBB Pro German Grand Prix (3rd Place)
1987	IFBB Pro French Grand Prix (3rd Place)
1988	IFBB Mr. Olympia (4th Place)
1988	IFBB Pro German Grand Prix (3rd Place)
1988	IFBB Pro Greek Grand Prix (1st Place)
1988	IFBB Pro British Grand Prix (1st Place)
1988	IFBB Pro Spanish Grand Prix, Madrid (1st Place)
1988	IFBB Pro Italian Grand Prix (2nd Place)
1988	IFBB Pro French Grand Prix (2nd Place)
1988	IFBB Pro Spanish Grand Prix, Barcelona (1st Place)
1989	IFBB Mr. Olympia (2nd Place)
1989	IFBB Pro Dutch Grand Prix (1st Place)
1989	IFBB Pro Finnish Grand Prix (1st Place)
1990	IFBB Mr. Olympia (2nd Place)
1991	IFBB Mr. Olympia (4th Place)
1992	IFBB Mr. Olympia (3rd Place)
1992	IFBB Pro World Cup (1st Place)
1993	IFBB Ironman Pro Invitational (2nd Place)
1993	IFBB Arnold Schwarzenegger Classic (2nd Place)
1993	IFBB Mr. Olympia (4th Place)

Are You Ready for the Next Step?

Congratulations on reading the Lean Body Promise. Twelve weeks from now you can be showing off the lean body you desire and deserve. And it all starts by entering **the 12-week Lean Body Challenge at www.leanbodypromise.com**

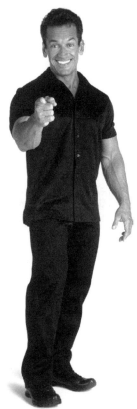

Dear Friend,

There's no feeling like the one you get when you make a positive change in your life. And there's no better way to change how you feel inside than by changing your body. Let's face it, when you look good, you feel good about yourself! Now's the time to make up your mind to release the lean body that's locked up inside you. And my 12-week online **Lean Body Challenge** is the perfect way to get yourself motivated to make it happen.

Once you sign up for the **Lean Body Challenge**, you'll begin receiving weekly encouragement and support from me, for the full twelve weeks. I'll send you helpful motivational tips by email every week to help you complete the challenge. With this support, you can't fail.

So now I ask you: Are you ready to get into the best shape of your life? If you can say, "Yes, I can do it!" with certainty, than you're ready to go. See you at the finish line.

Yours in health,

Lee Labrada

Lee Labrada

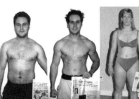

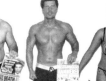
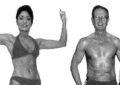